Prevention and Treatment of Sports Injuries

Anju Ambast

KHEL SAHITYA KENDRA
7/26, Ansari Road, Daryaganj,
New Delhi-110002

Published by:
KHEL SAHITYA KENDRA
7/26, Ansari Road, Darya Ganj, New Delhi-110002
Ph.: (O) 011-43551324, 42564726, 47090343
(M) 9811088729, (Fax) 011-42564726
(Res.) 47091605
E-mail: khelsahitya1@rediffmail.com
Web: www.khelsahitya.com, www.kskpublisher.com

ISBN 978-81-7524-264-7

PRINTED IN INDIA 2026

Printed by:
ASIAN OFFSET PRINTERS
Delhi

Laser Typesetting by:
K.S.K. DTP UNIT, DELHI

CONTENTS

Preface

Television and other media popularize the health fitness in general public. Now-a-days public of every age group are more conscious about their health. This public consciousness is responsible for mushroomious increase of gyms, health centers and sports clubs. Many untrained and unqualified persons are involved in this business. As well as many people are engaged in morning walk, evening walk, jogging and exercises on his own, without knowing the basic biomechanics of injuries, first aid and/ or preventive measures for injuries caused by these exercises. General physicians suggest not to do these exercises without under proper guidance.

Coaches or athletic trainer have a special role in the rehabilitation process because they are in an ideal position to maintain open and free communication with players and physicians. They are advisor and friend of the player, and eyes and ears of the physician. The importance of the coach as a key member of the sports team has become so obvious in competitions that every school who are seriously involve in sports, are having one coach as its staff member. Central role of the coaches in the sports team become due to their training not due to only their sports performance in national or state level tournaments.

The aim of this book is to give some glimpses of sports injuries for general population who are taking sports as a hobby as well as give some suggestions to fellow-athletes, coaches and physicians for treatment of the injured player. In Psychological Factors and Sports Injury author emphasizes the characteristics of injury prone athlete and coping strategy to overcome this trauma. By no means injuries relating to sports and exercise can be controlled. We can only minimize these injuries. In Prevention of Sports Injuries, preventive measures, in this regard, are described.

I would like to express my personal gratitude to the many people who made both obvious and subtle contributions to the development of this book.

First of all, I want to thank Dr. Ravi Ambast and Shri Anil Kumar for their valuable suggestions. Two chapter which are mentioned above are incorporated in this book only due to the suggestions received by them Without inclusion of these chapter this book might be left unbalanced.

My special thanks goes to my daughters, Richa and Rashi whose constant patience for love and affection help me to work on this book.

CHAPTER-1

BIOMECHANICAL PRINCIPLES OF INJURIES

The association between biological and mechanical aspects of movement has been said to give human motion its sophistication (Williams Sperryn, 1976). For this reason, the study of biomechanics has a direct application to injury and its recovery. Knowledge of this subject is essential for an understanding of the prevention, diagnosis and treatment of sports injuries.

Forces:

Force may be defined as a push or pull which produces or tends to produce a change in the state of rest or of uniform motion of a body or change the direction of motion of the body. The unit of measurement of a force is the Newton which is denoted by N. Newton is that force which acting on a mass of one kilogram produces an acceleration of one meter per second.

1 N = 1 Kg. x 1m/sec-2

Force applied on an object can do three things:

1. It can change the speed of the object making it move faster or slower,
2. It can change the direction of motion of the object, and
3. It can change the shape of the object.

NEWTON'S LAWS OF MOTION:

First law of motion is the law of intertia. It states that an object at rest or in uniform motion will remain at rest or in uniform motion unless an balanced force acts on it.

Intertia is the property or tendency of a body to resist any change in its state of rest or of uniform motion in a straight line.

If a body has a large intertia, it is hard to make it move. If a body with a large intertia is moving, it is hard to stop it or change its speed as well as its direction of motion.

In a strong kicking action, intertia will have to be overcome to start the limb moving. If the force required to do this is large and rapid encugh, muscle damage may occur.

As a result of its osteological formate and the properties of the joint structure, a joint has a certain intertia. Due to immobilisation the joint tissues will have stiffened and the joint fluid will have become more viscous, so the intertia is likely to be greater. Gentle and rhythmic swinging exercises are often used to mobilize stiff joints. The continuous motion is more effective than stopping, resting, and then starting again. In cases of severe weakness after injury, a muscle may be unable to overcome joint intertia to initiate movement.

The force of an object is proportional to the product of the mass of the object and its acceleration. It is the Newton's second law of motion.

When a football player kicks a football, the force with which he kicks, acts for the specific time that the leg is in contact with the football. The football has a certain mass and changes its velocity from that at the start to that at the finish of the action. It is known that momentum is the product of mass and velocity. Velocity at the start and at the finish is also known so the rate of change of this momentum can be obtained by dividing the difference in velocities by time.

Newton's third law states that in an interaction between two bodies the force exerted by the first body on the second is equal and opposite to that exerted by the second body on the first body.

When a player caught a forcibly coming ball, it is necessary to reduce its momentum to avoid injury. The aim of this act is to extend the time taken to dissipate the reaction force (Watkins, 1983). When ball is stopped with the arms and locked wrists, injury may occur due to sudden force. Injury risk may be reduced if the arms are extended to catch the ball and flexed as the ball is brought into the body. It is due to the extended time taken to dissipate the ball's force.

STRESS:

Mechanical stress is the force applied on the per unit area of an object. Three major categories of stress i.e. tension, compression and shear are important in sports injuries.

Tension: It is a pulling force, When the spine is flexed, the posterior spinal ligaments are tightened and resulted to a tension stress.

Compression: It is a push force which is opposite of tension. When the qauadriceps contract in a bent knee, the patella is pulled against the femur and compression stress is applied to the patello-femoral joint.

Shear: It occurs when opposite forces are applied to a tissue and one part of the tissue slide over another.

Fall on to the straight leg will result in compression stress on the joint structure. These forces will largely be absorbed but if severe, compression fracture may occur. If the joints bend during the fall, tension stress will be imposed on the muscles. Elasticity of the muscles will take some of the stress away from the joints. Stearing will occur between the body tissues, and foot and ground if anyone fall at an angle.

Relationship between Stress and Strain:

When a stress is applied to a tissue, the tissue will deform which is called strain. Strain is the result of interaction between stress and mechanical features of tissue. Some important mechanical features of tissue are stiffen, creep, fatigue, resilience, and toughness.

When a tissue is less elastic, structural stiffness occurs. When stress increases, less deformation occurs in the scar tissues. Scar tissue are stronger and less elastic in comparison to other tissues so will not respond to stress in the same manner.

When a load, especially small load, is laid on a material for a long time, creep occurs. This pressure deform the material very gradually. Creep is related with time so the degree of deformation is based on the amount of pressure applied to a tissue as well as the duration for which the pressure is applied. As a result, a lesser load applied over a greater time will produce a larger amount of creep.

Fatigue diminished productivity efficiency, or ability to carry on work, because of previous expenditure of energy in doing work.

Resilience is related with the ability of any material to absorb and release energy. This type of materials absorb energy well in the elastic range and return to the original shape when the stored energy is released.

Toughness is also related with the ability to absorb and release the energy. After the elasticity threshold, this type of materials burst quickly.

Lever Mechanism:

Lever is a long rigid rod, straight or bent which can turn about a support (fulcrum). The effort is applied at one end of the lever and the load is overcome on the other end. Effort tries to move the lever and the load tries to stop the movement.

The shortest distance between the line of action of the force or effort and the fulcrum is known as effort arm. The shortest distance between the line of action of the load or a resistance and the fulcrum is known as load-arm. The ratio of the effort arm to the load arm gives a value for the mechanical advantage. A small effort applied at a greater distance form the fulcrum is able to move a heavy load placed near the fulcrum.

Levers are divided into three types according to the position of the fulcrum, load and effort. In the first type of lever fulcrum is in between the effort applied and the load e.g. see-saw. In the second type of lever load is in between the fulcrum and the effort e.g. wheelbarrow. Effort is in between the fulcrum and the load, in the third type of lever e.g. forearm supporting a load.

This mechanism is useful in reducing the risk of injury. For example, lifting a 10 kg. weight is not dangerous. However lifting it at arms length in a bent over position with the legs straight will place excessive leverage on the spine, increasing the effect of the weight on the lumbar spine and making injury more likely.

Gravitation Theory:

Centre of gravity is the point at which all the weight of an object can be considered to act. In an object which is uniform in shape, e.g. ball, the centre of gravity will be at the centre of the object. But, with the heterogenous objects e.g. human body, this will be nearer to the larger and heavier end.

In the standing human body, centre of gravity is at S1/2 spinal level which will vary as the change in the position of body will take place. Centre of gravity is also determined by an objects weight so it will shift when we carry any object.

When we extend the centre of gravity in a line towards the floor, we can calculate the line of gravity. In order for any object to remain standing, its line of gravity must always pass through its base of support. When this line of gravity moves outside this area, the object will fall.

An object is more stable when its centre of gravity is lower. When the body becomes fatigued an unstable position is dangerous especially during the sports and physical exercises.

A wide base of support is more stable than slender base. For example an ice-skater skating on a line with thin blade of skate on the ice. His feet are close together so the base of support is very small. He is also standing straight which lift his centre of gravity. Combination of these two features makes him unstable. In contrast to this take an example of judo player. His feet wide apart has a wide base of support, his knees are bent lowering his centre of gravity and making him much more stable.

Form of Muscle:

Normally muscles may be classified according to the orientation of fibres. The fibres may be arranged in three fashion i.e. parallel obliquely and spiral. The arrangement of fibres determine the power and range of motion which the muscle can produce.

The first type of fibre arrangement is parallel. Here, the muscle fibres may be strap-like with individual fibres running the whole length of the muscle. Fibre arrangements may be either the sheet attaching to a broad flat tendon, or may be grouped into discrete bundles, producing a fusiform muscle belly which attaches to a tendon, or may run between adjacent tendinous intersections which divide the muscle as a whole into sections.

When the muscle fibres are attached to a central tendon, it is known as oblique grouping. In this grouping there are three alternatives for attachments of fibres to control tendon one, fibres may join to only one side of a tendon unipennate.

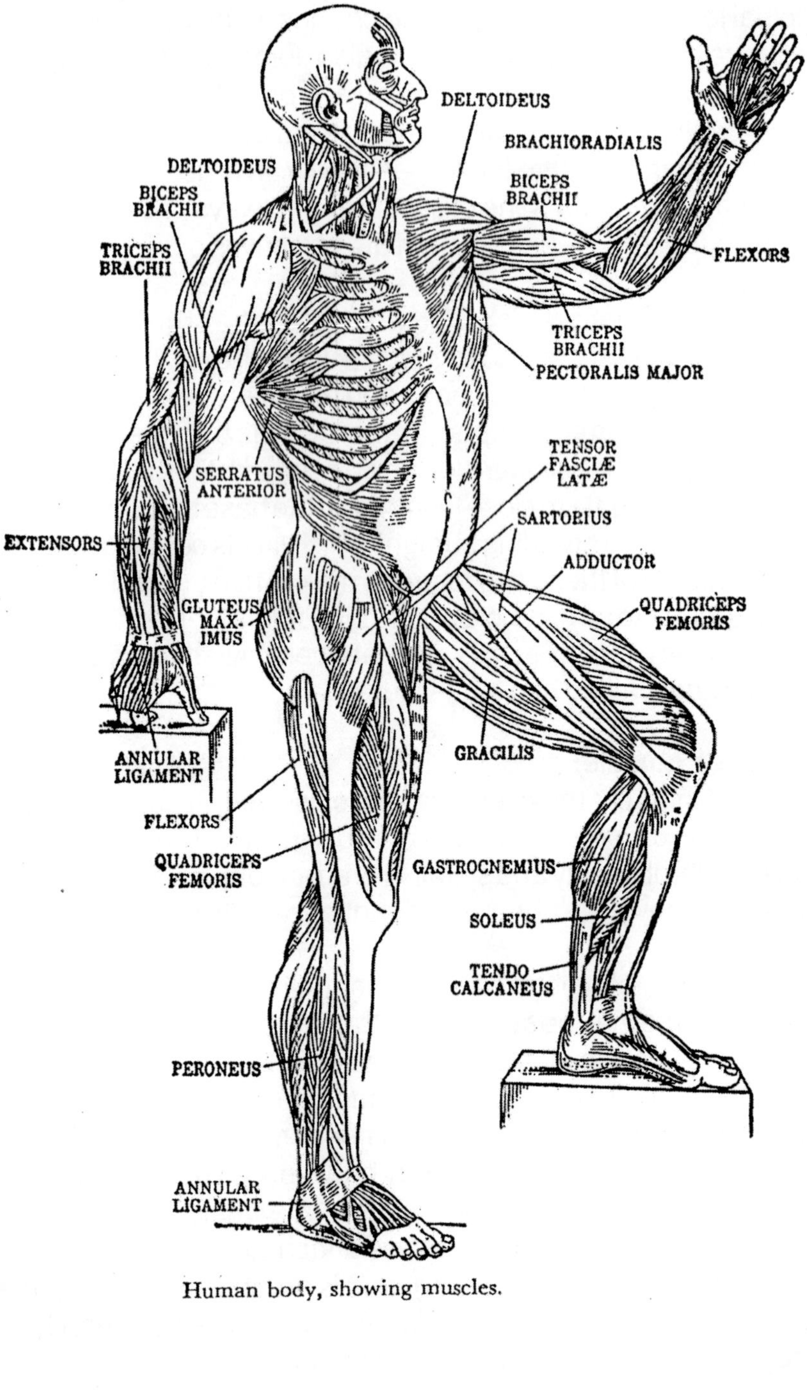

Human body, showing muscles.

Two, fibres find to both sides of a central septum (Bipennate). Three, muscle has several septa (Multipennate).

In spiralized type of fibre arrangement, muscle fibres twist as they travel between the two ends of the muscle.

Biomechanical Analysis:

Prevention and rehabilitation of sports injuries are only possible through the analysis of human movement. Observation is the basic technique for analysis but has a limitation by the visual memory of the observer. Although the trained and experienced observer may take considerable more data than the layman, precise analysis is not possible. Now through the video recording this task is much easier.

Recording of Movement:

With a view to record an action accurately, subject and his environment in which he performs must be pre-planned. Subjects should be suitably dressed to enable exact location of body segments and joints. Background should be clear and reference points of motion are marked on the skin with adhesive tape or coloured ink. Video camera should be set up on a stand at a set distance from the subject and should be capable of recording even in a poor lighting conditions. It should also have a timing / counting facility.

To minimize the distance error the distance from the camera to the subject must be remain the same, if two or more analyses are to be made. Synchorised camera placed at 90 degree to each other should be placed, if complex motions are to be recorded. The whole action should be recorded without moving the camera and the observer must be far enough away from the subject to get a wide field of view.

Analysis of the movement:

Analysis of a movement will be easily possible through slow down the action and use of an experienced analytical eye. Using this slow motion video picture mark various reference points. Now we may able to digitz the image and this will give a clear picture of total movement.

CHAPTER-2

PSYCHOLOGICAL FACTORS OF SPORTS INJURIES

A variety of psychological factors may predetermine an athlete to injury. Personality, anxiety, locus of control, self-esteem etc. are determining factors to injury received by any athlete. Several researches have attempted to show that specific aspects of personality make an athlete more prone to injury. In contrast, others argue that temporary mood states are more liable to have a significant effect on injury of an athlete.

Personality Profile Of Injury Prone Athlete:

Cattell's 16 PF test was used by many researchers on injured athletes and found that tender minded players were more likely to be injured, as well as, reserved and detached players suffered more severe injuries (Jackson, Jarrett, Bailey, Kausek, Swanson, & Powell, 1978). Reilly (1975) found a relationship between apprehensiveness and injury. He also opines that being over- protective, easily distracted, attention seeking may also prone to injury.

Sanderson (1981) has listed a number of psychological characteristics displayed by the injury-prone athletes .

1. Counter Phobia: Athlete attempts to counter anxiety by being overtly aggressive and fearless.
2. Sign of Masculinity: Athlete uses injury as a mark of courage. Continues to play despite injury, but exaggerates pain to seek admiration.
3. Masochism: Punishes oneself for feeling of guilt, often about failure to reach own unrealistic targets.
4. Injury as a Weapon: tries to punish others, for example, the young athlete who is forced to play by over zealous parents.
5. Escape: Athlete who fears competition because of feelings of inferiority, but cannot opt out for fear of isolation.

6. Psychosomatic injury: No physical injury or slight injury made worse by emotional factors.

When the manager..Bramwell Etal (1975) studied stressful life events as Life Change Units. Positive stressful life events included, marriage, getting a better job, passing an examination while negative events referred to divorce, failure in an examination. The results showed that injured players had significantly more Life Change Units in the one and two years preceding to injury, either in positive side or negative or in both sides. Risk of injury was five times greater when a major event (death of a parent, separation of parents etc.) had occurred (Coddingtons Troxell, 1980).

Kerr and Minden (1988) claimed that the majority of gymnasts reported `lack of concentration' and `thinking of other things' as the major cause of their injury. This lack of attention or concentration may be explained in the terms of psychological information processing system used by the athletes. Norris (1993) explains that skilled athletes rely on two information processing systems. One is allowing automatic or apparently effortless action which is faster and the other is slower and requires more conscious control. To perform well, an athlete must let go and allow these automatic actions to 'flow' freely. Any attempt to control the natural rhythm of the action will hinder its automatic naturel and result in a loss of efficiency. Stressful life events could lead to worry about perfomance, which in turn may prevent an athlete from letting go. Additionally, inappropriate thoughts may prevent the slower secondary system from monitoring overall performance efficiently. Stressful life events lead to mental fatigue which overtly shown as apathy.

After accepting the fact that an athlete is vulnerable to injury after a stressful life event, the training should be modified by reducing its intensity and concentrating on basic skills. A period of attention training to enable the athlete to focus on a task or to shift attention between different tasks rapidly, should be involved in training programme for this type of problematic athletes.

Reaction to Injury:

There are some definite stages of reactions of an athlete

to an injury. Primarily, injury is to be met with denial which turns into anger. After some time when athlete perceives the injury significant, he comes into the influence of depression. Finally when athlete overcomes the effect of depression, constructive attitude towards injury takes place which helps the rehabilitation process.

As per the responses of athletes to the injury, Gordon, Milios and Grove (1991) classified the behaviours of athletes during rehabilitation process which shows the positive and negative attitudes of athletes towards the injury.

Positive Behaviour:

Asks question to understand the injury.

Listens the advice of therapist.

Co-operation and compliance with therapist.

Receptive to restrictions placed on athlete.

Initiates rehabilitation instructions at home.

Early acceptance of injury.

Does not miss the appointments with the therapist.

Negative Behavior:

Failure to take responsibility for own rehabilitation.

Non-acceptance of injury.

Non-compliance and non-cooperation.

Denial of seriousness of injury.

Displays depression.

Bargaining with therapist over treatment and time out of competition.

Missing appointments.

As per the results of Anderson and William's (1988) studies, the rehabilitation process of the injury is influenced by many factors related to the athlete like personality, previous history of injury, level of competition and how serious the injury is perceived.

The level of competition and competitor are important in perception of injury Same injury give more loss to high level competitor in compression to low level competitor so the same injury will be perceived severe by the high level competitor in comparison to low level competitor.

Perception of the injury is also influenced by the nature of sports. The game like golf which is not physically demanding, to become injured is not socially acceptable. But in the other game, like football which is often perceived as a sign of manhood, same injury will be perceived severe.

Some parts of body produce greater psychological impact than others due to their actual or perceived utility in proper functioning of body. Injury to knee or back will be perceived seriously than the injury on other parts of body.

Personality and Reaction to Injury:

H.J. Eysenck (1957) has identified two major dimension of personality. First, the dimension of extraversion-introversion and secondly, a neureticism (instable-stable).

Extroverts are sociable, adventurous, talkative, frank and have open behaviour in dealing with others.

Introverts are hesitant, reflective and pessimistic.

Rehabilitation process is more boring to extroverts than introverts. Injury has greater psychological impact on introverts and they have lower tolerance of pain. During rehabilitation process these athletes need strong encouragement.

Stable athletes (introvert or extrovert) are calm, even tempered, emotionally stable and less problematic.

The highly instable or neurotic athletes are more nervous, mood and anxious so they are hard to deal with. As the extroverts have a strong self-esteem, so the neurotic extroverts will often perceive their self-esteem to be threatened by injury and emotional problems may occur. The neurotic-introverts are more likely to develop phobias and anxiety (Sanderson 1977).

Psychological Aspects of Pain:

A level at which a person describes actually the feeling of a stimulus which is called sensory threshold, is roughly the same for everyone but pain threshold is influenced by individual and cultural differences. Both the differences are influenced by a wide variety of psychological factors. Personality, life style, habits, cultural and religious differences influence pain tolerance.

Extroverts have higher pain threshold than introverts due

to cortical inhibition (Eysenck, 1967). Extroverts tend to express pain more freely and are more ready to accept social disapproval occurred due to this pain or injury (Griffiths, 1980).

The situation is important in which the person experiences the pain. Injured soldiers requested less morphine than civilians (Beecher, 1959). In the same way, boxers are often not noticed the injuries, because their attention is focused elsewhere.

Individual's past history and understanding the causes of pain are also relevant for pain perception. Through learning process we learn how to respond to a painful stimulus. When a person understands the cause of his pain, anxiety will reduce and pain intensity will also lowered otherwise he tends to complain more pain.

During illness the body's sensory awareness may be lowered, and positive emotions can help to restore the normal pain. In the rehabilitation process, physiotherapist may affect the intensity and meaning of the athletes pain, both negatively and positively. He can change athlete's attitude towards pain which can make the athlete a `pain manager' ratherthan `pain victim'. Athletes should encouraged to participate in controlled exercise and recreational activities rather than to suffer chronic pain. As per Williams (1989) study, combining fear reduction with confidence building about 80% of patients given up illness symptom.

Motivation:

Motivation leads an individual to engage in and /or sustain, a particular activity. Motivation fulfils a need in an athlete and that need will change with time. We must recognize the athletes' need which helps to motivate athlete's to perform a particular task.

Motivating factors may be personal- social and intrinsic-extrinsic. Social and personal factors will merge to change the meaning of a situation which an athlete has. It will also help to determine the behaviour such as effort, persistence and performance. In the same way, motivation must consist of a combination of both intrinsic and exterimsic rewards. This combination should be carefully plannec.

Lewthwaite (1990) recognized three personal motivational factors, including both intrinsic and extrinsic rewards, which are important in the context of exercise and injury. These are goal-setting, belief of one's personal capability and perceptual affective experience.

Goal setting:

Generally, two types of goals are used in sports. The first is task involved goal and the second is ego-involved goal. The first rely on the need to improve a skill or performance and the second one focus on the necessity to prove oneself and be judged as competent or atleast avoid being judged incompetent.

Goals are also based on time. In the context of time scale, goals may be either long term or short term. Long-term goals are the things an athlete wants to achieve as the end result of training or rehabilitation. In contrast short term goals are those which the athlete wants immediately and will affect one's immediate performance.

When an athlete is instrumental in the goal setting process, goals will be set to a higher standard. Several researches have described the benefits of goal setting in respect to the performance of the athlete. Locke and Bryan (1966) and Harari (1969) showed specific goals to be better to general goal because specific goal group not only performed better but had a faster rate of performance improvement. A number of features are important in the goal setting process. A goal should be:

1. Specific: For example specify a set number of repetitions or weight to be lifted rather than to say 'do your best'.
2. Meaningful: Give a reason for obtaining the goal to the athlete.
3. Difficult: Goal should be difficult enough to stretch an athlete.
4. Obtainable: Goal should be achievable because failure to achieve a short term goal over a number of trials will develop frustration.
5. Measurable: One must know if he is achieving the goal or not.
6. Individual: Previous performance and individual factors should be taken into consideration to set the goal.
7. Participation: Athlete's participation in the goal making process is more effective.

Belief in Capability:

Bandura (1982) pointed out two types of self-confidence.

First, efficacy expectation. It is the belief of a person that he can achieve something because of his innate abilities. Second, outcome expectations. It is the belief that when one acts in a particular manner, a particular result will follow.

Using this theory in the field of sports injury rehabilitation, it is not enough for an athlete undergoing rehabilitation to believe that a certain flexibility exercise will restore full range of movement. He must also be encouraged to believe that he has the capability to bear discomfort and to persist with the exercise programme.

Perceptual- Affective Experience:

Self perception of one's effort and the emotion attached to that effort can act as a motivation. People tend to resist with uncomfortable or painful actions but tend to persist with activities which are enjoyable. There is an individual difference in what is enjoyable and what is painful.

It is more likely that an athlete will work hard in an enjoyable group atmosphere in contrast to a training session with full of begrudge because social context and the emotions attached to an exercise can act as a motivator.

Addiction is a process rather than a condition. Individuals can indeed become addicted to exercise, just as they can become addicted to drugs, smoking, meditation or television.

These withdrawal symptoms include, anxiety, restlessness, guilt, irritability, tension, bloatedness, muscle twitching and discomfort.

Exercise Addiction:

As per Crossman etl (1987) the experience of exercise for an athlete is one factor which determine whether an exercise become addictive or not. Addiction is a process rather than a condition. Individuals can indeed become addicted to exercise just as they can become addicted to drugs, smoking, meditation or television. Addiction reflects the athlete's need for exercise which is either physiological or psychological. The addiction can be positive or negative. Positive addiction reflects that an athlete receives some psychological or physical benefit from an activity and is able to control that activity. But negatively addicted athlete is controlled by the activity. They will also experience severe negative affects or withdrawal symptoms with a missed part of exercise. These withdrawal syptoms include anxiety, restlessness, guilt, initability, tension, bloatedness, muscle twitching and discomfort. This type of athlete often exercises alone or in isolation from the group and fails to gain approval from the significant others.

Some important characteristic of exercise addicted athlete are as under:

1. In order to complete an exercise the athlete tend to ignore physical discomfort or injury.
2. Exercise addicted athletes exercise alone or isolate themselves in a group setting.
3. This type of athletes perform several trials of exercise in contrast to non-addicted athletes.
4. Exercise gives him high satisfaction and less self-criticism.
5. After missing any set of exercise, he may be more depressed, anxious and angry.

CHAPTER-3

HEAD AND CERVICAL SPINE INJURIES

The central nervous system (brain and spinal cord) is unique because the nerve cells are incapable of regeneration. Cells of these body parts that die are forever lost, incapable of replacement with artificial hardware, transplantation or regrowith; while other major joints like knee, hip, ankle, elbow and other body organs have the capacity of replacement. The central nervous system place in the skull and spine is the sole organ where this is not possible.

Several important and simultaneous observations must be made, whenever sports person fell unconscious due to injury. This observation include blood pressure, pulse, respiratory rate, state of consciousness, pupillary size and reactivity.

Subsequent evaluation and treatment is dependent upon this initial examination. If within a few minutes there is an improvement in the condition of the patient, then subsequent transportation and diagnostic evaluation can be proceeded . If any kind of deterioration in the state of consciousness is seen, transportation and treatment must be precipitous. Fracture board should be used for transportation of the unconscious injured player. Head of that player should be secured in a neutral position with sand bags, a four-poster collar or a traction device, which is available.

The helmet can be used as an instrument for cervical fracture. The chin strap serves as a halter and the ear holes or adjacent edge of the helmet serves as a site for attachment of neutral traction. If an unconscious player is wearing a helmet with good airways, helmet should not be removed. If the airway is a questionable, helmet should be removed with some precautions like, don't remove the helmet with force and during removal of the helmet neck should be in a neutral position (neither flexed nor extended).

If the fracture board is not readily available to transport the unconscious player, a decision must be taken whether to wait to the ambulance or transport the player using the locked-arm technique. If an adequate number of players or spectators are available, by locking the hands to the elbows of individuals standing opposite each other, a secure surface for transporting the injured player a short distance is provided.

Sports Risky for Head and Cervical Spine:

Motor cycle racing, football, diving, automobile racing and hand gliding have maximum risk to head and cervical spine. Gymnastics, horse riding, mountaineering, parachuting, ski jumping, sky gliding and sky diving are the sports with high risk for head and cervical spine. According to Bodnar (1977) in automobile racing during their initial two years 30 percent of new participants were either killed or so seriously injured that they could not compete again. Motor cycles are even more dangerous.

Eighty percent of the serious injuries befall those who have been riding for six months or less. Hang gliding ranks at the top in reference of serious injuries or fatalities.

Head Injuries

1. Concussion: Most common head injury in sports is concussion. It is in three types, first defined as a fleeting alteration of brain function, with a period of unconsciousness, and then complete brain recovery. Many concussions occur without a lapse in consciousness. It is a very mild form of concussion in which there is no loss of consciousness but only lapse of memory after the head trauma. Many boxers and football players face this type of problem.

In the severe form of concussion, one is unconscious transiently; and in more severe form of concussion, one is unconscious for a more prolonged time. In these instances, the head trauma causes alterations in the functions of the reticular activating system, which runs from the upper cervical spinal cord to the thalamus. This results in unconsciousness, changes in pulse rate, respiration and blood pressure. As the reticular activating system functions properly, all the other related disabili-

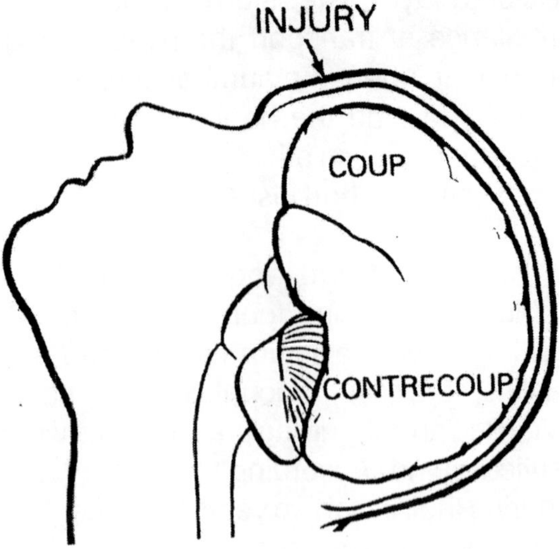
INJURY
COUP
CONTRECOUP

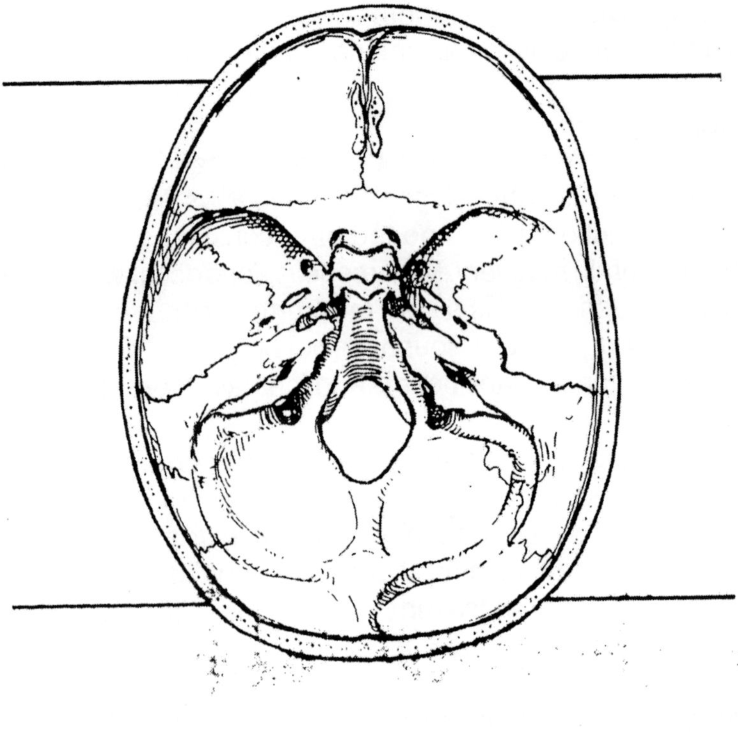

ties resume normal function.

Degree and duration of amnesia (memory loss) are positively related with the severity of the concussion (brain injury). In the mild brain injury, memory loss is usually only for events immediately after the head trauma. But in the severe brain injury player may lost the memory of that event. In severe brain injury, player should be removed from the game and some medical examination should be done followed with the placement in a medical facility for 24 hours of neurologic observation. In minor brain injury in certain instances where the player is fully lucid with no headache, return to play is permissible but he should be observed closely over the next 24 hours in case blood clot is developing. This player should be under no circumstances allowed to be left alone that first night and awakened every two hours during the night.

If the player got two brain injury of severe nature in a short span of time, it is generally agreed that the player should not be allowed to participate in the competition for some time, particularly for that season.

When the player is free from headache and has a normal EEG (electroencephalograph) he may safely resume competition. Before giving this permission, a thorough review of circumstances resulting in the brain injury should be conducted. In this review few basic points may be determined like (a) if the player was using his head unwisely, illegally or both (b) if the player was wearing the equipment correctly, and (c) the equipment itself should be rechecked to be certain that it not only is worn properly but fits correctly as well.

2. Intracranial Hemorrhage: It is a leading cause of death from athletic head injury. Intracranial hemorrhage is of four types and all the four types may be fatal so rapid accurate initial assessment as well as appropriate follow up is mandatory.

The first type is called extradural hematoma which is frequently associated with a fracture of the temporal home and results from a tear in one of the arteries supplying the covering of the brain. It accumulates inside the skull but outside the covering (dura) of the brain. Any functional or structural damage in brain by this injury sometime progress rapidly and reach a fatal size in 30

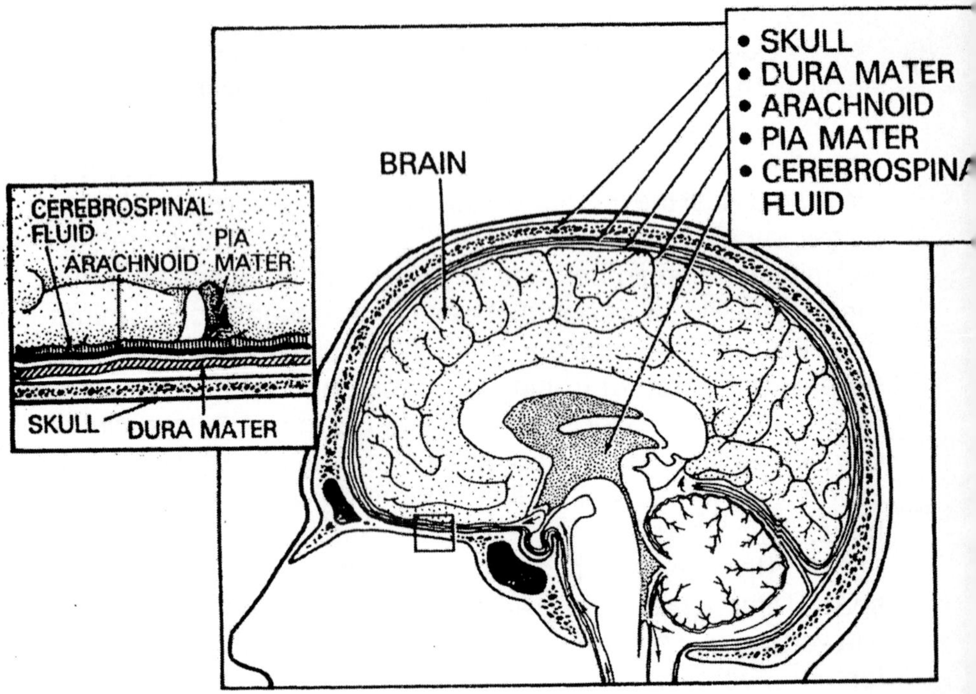
• SKULL
• DURA MATER
• ARACHNOID
• PIA MATER
• CEREBROSPINAL FLUID
BRAIN
CEREBROSPINAL FLUID
ARACHNOID
PIA MATER
SKULL
DURA MATER

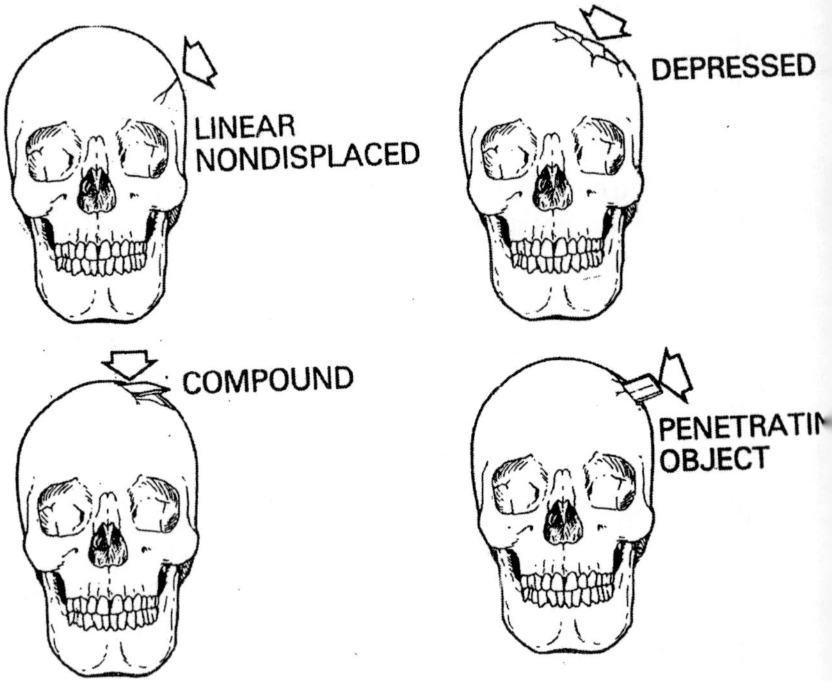
LINEAR NONDISPLACED
DEPRESSED
COMPOUND
PENETRATIN
OBJECT

to 60 minutes and sometimes it takes one to two hour. Initially the player may regain consciousness after the head trauma and before starting to experience increasing headache and deterioration in the consciousness as the clot accumulates and the intracranial pressure increases, there is sufficient time for medical help. Normally the brain is free from direct injury. If the clot is removed surgically without loss of time, full recovery may be achieved. This type of injured player should be kept in intensive care for the next 24 hours at the place where full neurosurgical services are immediately available.

A second type of intracranial hemorrhage occurs between the brain surface and the dura, and called subdural hematoma. It results either from a torn vein running from the surface of the brain to the dura, or from a torn venous sinus or even a small artery on the surface of the brain. In subdural hematoma, the player usually does not regain consciousness and immediate neurosurgical treatment is necessary. If this surgery is done within 24 hours of injury, blood clotting and associated brain damage may be minimized and the life of the player may be saved. Sometimes, the brain itself may not be injured but after few days or weeks a subdural hematoma may develop. This chronic subdural hematoma often associated with headache and cause a variety of mild or imperceptible mental motor or sensory symptoms. This type of damage will be detected through computerized axial tomography (CAT) scan.

A third type of intracranial hemorrhage is called intracerebral hematoma in which the bleeding is into the brain itself from a torm artery. Rapture of a congenital vascular lesion such as an aneurysm or arteriovenous malformation may also result in the form of intracerebral hematoma. It is very severe form of injury in which death occasionally occurs before the injured player can be moved to a hospital.

Fourth type is known as subarachnoid, confined to the surface of the brain. According to the Cantu (1987) following head trauma, such bleeding is the result of disruption of the tiny surface brain vessels and is analogous to a bruise. Since bleeding is superficial, surgery is not usually required unless a congenital vascular anomaly is present.

Cervical Spine Injuries:

Traumatic lesions that affect cervical spinal cord is same as it affects the brain like concussion and the various types of hemorrhages. The major concern with a cervical spine injury is the possibility of an unstable fracture that may produce the paralysis of arms and legs (quadriplegia). Without taking the X-rays, it is impossible to determine the presence of unstable fracture. A cervical cord injury or cervical fracture is usually synchronsed by rigid cervical muscle spasm and pain only if the player is fully conscious. It will indicate the presence of unstable fracture. Unconscious player is unable to say about the neck hurts. His neck muscles are also not in protective spasm. So no neck manipulation be carried out on the field and all the precautions must be followed which are discussed earlier in this chapter.

In addition to the afore said neck injuries other deformities may occur including stretch or traction injury to the brachial plexus or a nerve root. This condition either results from a forceful blow to the head from the side, or from head extension or from depression of the shoulder while the head and neck are fixed. In this injury player feels a shocklike sensation of pain and numbness radiating into the arm and hand. If the player receives this type of injury repeatedly over a period of years, it may lead weakness of the major muscles as well as constant pain. Some precaution like use of high cervical collar which controls neck flexion and extension, changing the player's hitting technique or changing the player's position in the field, may eliminate the problem.

An uncommon but very serious neck injury involves the carotid arteries. By either extremes of lateral flexion or extension or a forceful blow by a relatively fixed, narrow object impaling one's neck in a forward fall, the inner layer of the carotid may be torn. It can lead to clot formation at the site of injury and resulting in emboli to the brain or a complete occlusion of the artery (Cantu, 1987).

How to prevent head and cervical spine injuries:

With the use of appropriate protective headgaurd, we may limit the head injuries in large proportion. Initially, brain cannot be trained to accept the trauma of the injury but once the brain is injured, it is more sensitive for future injury.

In contrast to the brain, neck can be strengthened through training and exercise, to reduce the injury risk. Four movements of the neck i.e. flexion, extension, lateral bending and rotation, can be strengthened with the help of machines as well as using the resistance of other player's wrist.

Most serious neck injuries occur in diving, performed without any proper supervision. Following tips suggested by Shields etal (1978) may minimize the neck injury:

1. Never dive in unfamiliar water.
2. Be sure that the water is deep enough for diving. Familiar lakes and rivers change their levels.
3. If you are present when a spinal cord injury occurs, keep the victim's head and neck from bending and twisting.
4. Never dive near construction work because water level may have dropped, and dangerous objects may be just beneath the surface.
5. Alcohol distorts judgement so do not use alcohol before diving or swimming.
6. Water around the raft can be dangerous, especially if the water level is down. A slackened cale permits the raft to drift, putting the cable and anchor into the diving area.
7. Cloudy water can conceal hazardous objects. Before diving or swimming check the bottom.

Cantu (1987) in his article gave guideline to indicate when an athlete with a head or neck injury should be removed from a contest, kept out for the remainder of a season, or recommended never to return to contact sports competition.

A. Conditions that require removal from the remainder of the contest:

1. Concussion with residual effects (retrograde amnesia, confusion, headache, unexplained behaviour).
2. Pinched nerve (branchial plexus injury) in which there is a question about the possibility of a cervical spine injury.

A thorough re-examination must be conducted before the player is allowed to resume practice or competition.

B. Conditions that require discontinuation of contact sports for the remainder of the season:

1. Seizure secondary to head trauma, single or multiple, focal or generalized. Particular attention must be paid to the determination of the etiology in order to exclude any pre-existing cerebral abnormality.
2. Brachial plexus injury producing significant neurologic impairment.
3. Ruptured intervertebral disc, with or without surgery.
4. Prolonged post- concussion syndrome.

C. Conditions that absolutely contraindicate contact sports competition:

1. Symptomatic neurologic or pain-producing abnormalities about the foramen magnum.
2. Congenital spinal anomaly with potential instability that would render the spinal cord vulnerable.
3. Temporary quadriplegia, regardless of the etiology or the degree of recovery.
4. Spinal cord abnormalities, e.g. syringomyelia, arteriovenous malfunction.
5. Permanent central neurologic seguelal from head injury, e.g. organic dementia, homonymous hemianopsia.
6. Spontaneous subarachnoid hemorrhage from any cause.
7. Cervicomeduallary-vascular injury, with or without recovery.

CHAPTER-4

INJURIES TO THE SHOULDER AND ELBOW

Now a days shoulder and elbow injuries are common. When player complains of shoulder pain, the first step to diagnose the injury, is to determine whether the injury was a contact or non contact type of injury. Most injuries to the shoulder are the soft tissue type. This soft tissue injuries occur in the musculotendinous units of the shoulder and elbow. Especially in the case of throwing games. These injuries occur from over use and the poor bio-mechanics.

Rest, anti-inflammatory medications, stretching and strengthening exercise respond well, if early diagnosis is made. As the injuries become chronic, weakness and progressive loss of function may be detected.

SHOULDER INJURIES

For treatment of this type of injury, pain pattern, character, duration and eliciting factors need to be evaluated. A dull aching problem, normally at night, corresponds with rotator cuff tears; whereas burning pain is more typical of bursitis or tendinitis.

Knowledge of location of pain is very important for diagnostic purposes. Pain over the acromioclavicular joint might suggest degenerative disease and if associated with trauma, the physician should suspect an acromioclavicular joint sprin. If the pain is deep in the shoulder, it may come from rotator cuff involvement, synovitis, or glenoid labrum tear.

Like knowledge of location of pain, knowledge of the phase of the throwing motion during which the symptoms occur, is also essential. According to Andrews and Gillogly (1985) a popping or catching noise inside the joints often indicates a glenoid labrum tear. In general, dislocation is caused by a contact injury but subluxation anteriorly or poster iorly can be caused by contact or non-contact injuries. If the stability of the shoulder is affected by trauma or fatigue, such intra-articular structures as the labrum can be torn by traction of the biceps tendon or impingement between the humeral head and glenoid cavity.

Main injuries in regard to shoulder are acromioclavicular injury, shoulder subluxation or dislocation and rotator cuff injury.

1. Acromioclavicular Injury:

The mechanism of this type of injury is direct force onto the point of the shoulder, resulting in a sprain and sometimes a fracture of the distal clavicle. Sprain either involves capsular and ligamentous stretching without frank disruption (grade I) or rupture the capsule and acromioclavicular ligament (grade II) or disrupt both the acromioclavicular and coracoclavicular ligaments causing tenderness and swelling along the ligaments (grade III). X-ray films of grade II injury reveal slight elevation of the clavicle when compared to the uninvolved side. According to Happenstall (1975) X-ray films with 10 pound weights in the hands for grade III injury reveal upward drift of the distal clavicle on the involved side. For assessing a grade III acromioclavicular joint sprain Bearden etl (1973) suggest that the coracoclavicular distance should be more than 1.3 cm.

Grade I and II acromioclavicular joint sprain normally react well to immobilization in a sling and ice. After disappearance of pain, rehabilitation process should be started which give good results. Treatment of grade III sprains is controversial. Some physicians find surgery for best result and some find non surgical treatment as effective as surgical treatment. It is upto the player and the physician which treatment they want to use.

2. Shoulder subluxatilion and dislocation:

Subluxation occurs when the humeral head slips over the glenoid rim and then relocates spontaneously whereas dislocation occurs when the humeral head loses contact with the glenoid and lodges along the side of the joint. According to Rowe and Zarins (1981) subluxation can be so transient that the athlete only feels a sudden pain and the arm `goes dead'. It may occur without contact in the throwing athlete. Rowe and Zarins (1982) stated that in posterior dislocation, the arm is locked in internal rotation and the athlete is unable to externally rotate the arm, whereas in anterior dislocation the athlete is unable to internally rotate the arm and can not touch the opposite shoulder with the hand of the involved arm. Both the dislocations are diagnosed with the help of X-ray.

Simonet and Cofield (1984) recommended three to six weeks of immobilization in a sling succeeded by an intensive rehabilitation programme of muscular strengthening exercises with special emphasis on the internal rotator muscles for dislocation and the same exercise for at least six weeks in the case of subluxation.

3. Rotator Cuff Injury: In a throwing athlete, the labrum is more commonly damaged during the acceleration phase of the throwing act. It may damage labrum anteriorly as well as superiorly. During this movement, the horizontal adduction and internal rotation places a grinding force on the labrum. If the posterior stabilizing muscles are weak, the anterior force may succeed in damaging the labrum (Mcleod, 1985).

Tears of rotator cuff are frequently evident in the thrower's shoulder. It is the result of repeated microtrauma to the supraspinatus tendon. The biomechanical fault is in the deceleration stage, as weak posterior rotator cuff muscles attempt to restrain the forward movement of the humerus. Rotator cuff tear is more frequently seen in middle-aged males. The partial tear causes pain in the shoulder whereas complete tear usually results in a loss of active abduction beyond the first 30 degrees and passive abduction remains full (Booth & Marvel, 1975).

Shoulder movement and exercises are more effective treatment for rotator cuff injuries. Complete rest in a sling will often add another complications. So, anti-inflammatory medication, rest, and strengthening and flexibility exercises are the most important elements of treatment for rotator cuff injuries.

If we do not find positive results from the above treatment within six weeks, we may use arthroscopic surgery for this injury.

ELBOW INJURIES

The primary purpose of the shoulder may be described as

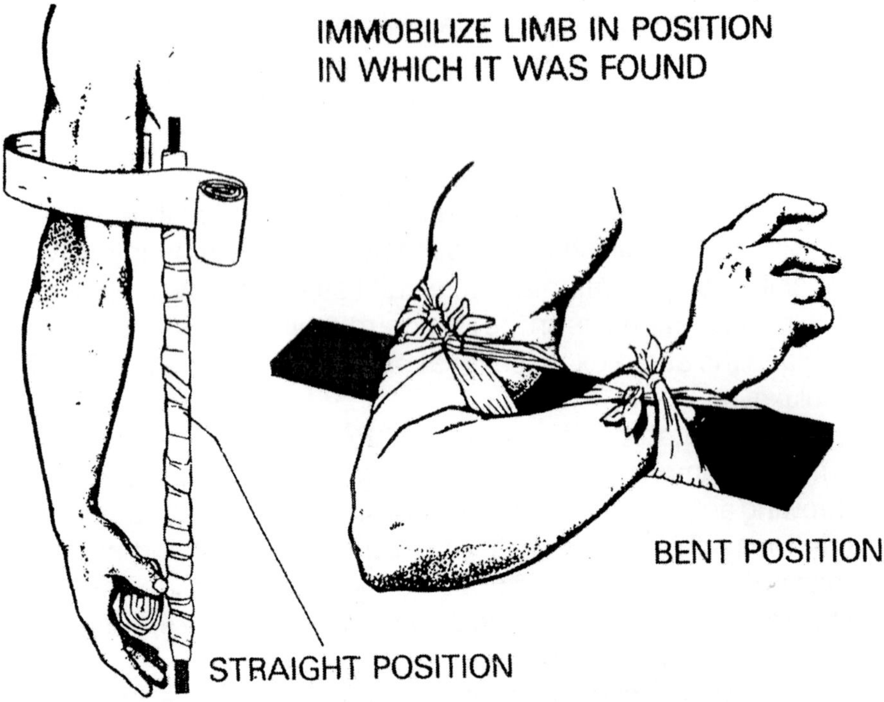

positioning the arm to facilitate hand action but the elbow functions to shorten or lengthen the arm, largely to allow the hand to be brought to the mouth. The elbow complex consists of humero-radial and humero-ulnar articulations and the superior radioulnar joint, all of which share the same capsule. Elbow and wrist are so connected with each other that any traumatic injury to the elbow is therefore likely to affect the wrist and to be a complete a clinincal examination should include both joint.

1. Lateral Pain:

Lateral epicondylitis normally presents as pain over the region of the lateral epicondyle, extending distally. The pain may build up slowly due to overuse or may be the result of a single incident. In general, pain is increased with resisted wrist extension. Depending on the site of the damage, pain can be made worse by adding forearm supination and redial deviation of the wrist. Performing resisted wrist extension with the elbow fully extended will usually elicit pain even in mild cases.

The primary site of the damage of lateral epicondylitis is the tendon of extensor carpi radialis brevis . In some cases, the extension carpadialis longus is affected at its attachment to the suprtacondylar ridge, and in some cases the front portion of the extensor digitorum. In general, the injury is at the temoperiosteal junction but scar tissue may form on the tendon itself, or on the musculotendinous junction. After repetition of the activity, granulated tissue may be formed on the underside of the tendon unit and at the tenoperiosteal junction. The major problem is that the granulation tissue does not progress quickly to a mature form, so healing fails to take place.

2. Medial Pain:

Medial side of the joint normally suffer due to throwing action. The throwing action imposes a number of stresses on the elbow. One of the throwing technique which affects this joint can be as stated: First, the shoulder is abducted and taken into extreme extemal rotation and extension while the elbow remains flexed. Then the shoulder and trunk rapidly move forward, leaving the arm behind. By this action there are more stress on the joint and stretches the ulnar collateral ligament. There are contraction between shoulder flexors and intemal rotators which fling the arm forward resulting in stress to the olecranon as the arm extends rapidly to full range.

3. Posterior Elbow Pain:

Pain at the back of the elbow is common in sports including throwing sports, and punching in martial art because these sports rapidly extend or hyperextend the joint. In these games structures involved are insertion of the triceps and the olecranon bursa, either individually or in combination.

The olecranon bursa is placed at the bony point of the elbow, over the inner-most olecranon process. Sometimes a deeper bursa is present between the capsule and triceps. The bursa can become inflamed either by leaming on the elbow for a prolonged period or due to a direct fall onto the point of the elbow. The second situation may induce hemorrhage into the bursal sac itself. In this case there is no abnormality in the joint but pain and thickening occur to direct palpation over the bursa.

Repeated strain on the triceps may cause inflammation of the triceps tendon with damage to the muscultoendinous or teno-osseous junction.

4. Muscular Injury:

The biceps, triceps and brachialis may be injured in many sports. The most common injury for the biceps is to its long head as well as its lower insertion. If only resisted flexion is painful but supination is not painful, the brachialis is indicated. In this situation the site of the pain is the centre of the front of the arm and in severe case the site of the pain is the wrist of the injured player.

In the case of injury to the triceps, the main site is musculotendinous junction. Clinical sign of this injury is the pain on resisted elbow extension but if this pain is felt in the upper arm nearer to the shoulder, the pain may be from the impingement of a shoulder structure.

5. Elbow Dislocation:

The prime sports which cause elbow dislocation are horse-riding, cycling, gymnastic, roller skating because the athlete usually falls backwards onto an abducted straight arm. There is often a crack at the time of injury with immediate swelling.

Treatment of lateral and medial epicondylitis entres around rest from the activity, anti-inflammatiories, and specific flexibility and strengthening exercises for the flexors and extensors of the wrist. If there is no positive result from this treatment, a steroid and local anesthetic injection and elbow splint may be helpful. Manual therapy, including local massage to reduce swelling and produce hyperaemia, and transverse frictions to form a mobile scar, are both of use. It is important to locate the exact site of injury for transverse frictions to be effective.

In the case of elbow dislocation, if the arm is immobilized for more than a week, the resting position should be in as much extension as possible (Garrick and Webb, 1990). It is important because reduced flexion is far easier to regain during rehabilitation than is extension. Gentle isometric exercise may be used as pain and swelling settles, except in case of complicated injury and after 2-3 days active mobility exercise is started with caution in the pain free range. According to Mehlhoff et al (1988) early mobilization of this injury is essential. Inactiveness for longer period showed poor results.

CHAPTER-5

ANKLE AND SPECIFIC INJURIES

Ankle is very important body part for transmission of body weight during running or walking. It is capable of the adjustments necessary for time balance on a wide variety of the surface. It is often involved in static and dynamic deformities that normally do not affect other parts of body because the joint is subject to the concentrated stress associated with standing as well as movement. The prevalence of ankle injury has been estimated by Connolly (1981) as at least one significant ankle sprain per day per 10,000 population. A casual approach to the diagnosis and treatment of these injuries is not logical because ankle injuries are not always minor. These are also associated with prolonged disability and recurrent instability for several months to several years.

Mechanism and anatomy of ankle joint:

The ankle joint consists of the trochlea surface of the talus and the distal ends of the tibia and fibula. The talar trochlea is wider anteriorly, and so plantarflexion is more free than dorsiflexion, average values being 30-50 degree and 20-30 degree respectively (Palastanga, Field and Soames, 1989). Marked variations occur both between individuals and following injury, and normal foot function can be achieved with as little as 20 degree of plantarflexion and 10 degree of dorsiflexion (McPoil and Brocato, 1990). Greater amounts of dorsiflexion are required as running speed or stride length increase.

The ankle is essentially a hinge, externally rotated to 20-25 degree with the malleoli. In the neutral position, with the foot perpendicular to the lower leg, there is very little frontal or transverse plane motion. With dorsiflexion, abduction of the foot is possible, and during plantarflex on, adduction can occur. In dorsiflextion the broad anterior par: of the talus is forced into the narrower mortice between the tibia and fibula. The interosseous and transverse tibiofibular ligaments are stressed, as the bones and the joint moves into close pack position.

Plantarflexion sees the narrow posterior part of the trochlear surface of the talus moving into the broader tibio-fibuldar mortice.

Recoil of the above ligaments causes the malleoli to approximate and maintain contact with the talus.

The ankle joint is strengthened by a variety of ligaments. In regard to the injury, collateral ligament is the important one. Both collateral ligaments- medial and lateral travel from the malleoli and have bands attaching to the calcaneus and talus.

The larger and stronger deltoid ligament is fan shaped, arises from the medial malleolus, and inserts on the navicular, calcaneal and talar bones. The medial ligament has both superficial and deep components. Superficial components are tibiotalar, tibiocalcaneal and tibionavicular; and deep component is posterior talotibial. The ligament particularly the latter component, stablises the joint during eversion and prevents subluxation. There are three distinct lateral collateral ligaments. The anterior talofibular ligament arises from the anterior tip of the fibula and attaches to the lateral neck of the talus. Its function is to prevent anterior and lateral subluxation of the talus during plantar flexion. Running from the fibula tip to the lateral aspect of the calcaneus in the posteroinferior direction is the calcaneal fibular ligament. This ligament functions to prevent lateral subluxation of the talus during strong adduction of the calcaneus. The posterior talofibular ligament arises from the posterior aspect of the lateral malleolus and inserts on the posterolateral margin of the talus as the strongest of the three lateral collateral ligaments. It is responsible for preventing posterior subluxation of the talus during forced dorsiflexion.

Field Management and Rehabilitation:

Time lapse between injury and the subsequent evaluation of the ankle injury is very crucial. Normally, athletes perceived majority of injuries as mild. They do not take any medical assistance for many days, until the amount of swelling, functional disability and spasm are maximum. Initial 20 to 30 minutes of injury are golden period for the purpose of evaluation. There is no discoloration, swelling and disability during this period. Before diffuse swelling, discoloration and experience of acute pain, evaluation of an injury through palpation will be extremely valuable in eliciting point tenderness. These discomforts prohibit visual identification of the precise location of injury. Injured ankle should be compared with the uninjured side in order to estimate deviation from normal ligament tightness. Active and passive range of motion should be evaluated after inspection and palpation.

For all type of acute ankle injuries, immediate treatment consists of rest, ice, immobilization, compression and elevation. For the first 24 hours ice should be applied on the injury for 15-20 minutes with the gap of about two hours. Ice should not be kept directly on the skin. Plastic bags should be used for this purpose. Adhesive surgical tape, posterior splint made from fibreglass or plaster of paris may give best result for immobilization. Cream (1981) has suggested on the basis of his study that a 24-hour period of immobilization and compression folowed by rapid mobilization will achieve full functional mobility in 99% of patients in two weeks with soft tissue injuries.

To give suggestion regarding return of injured player to play is perhaps the most difficult area for a team physician. In general, one player should not be allowed to return to play until the range of motion and strength of the injured ankle is equal to that of the un-injured ankle. In an emergency case only those players who are with the mildest ankle injuries i.e. no pain, no spasm and no functional disability, should be allowed to return for play with the precaution that the ankle is to be taped and cryotherapy regularly applied during rest periods. In case of severe injuries or injuries that have not been completely evaluated, the player should be removed from the game.

In the sub-acute phase, massage, especially, finger kneading around the malleolus is of value in preventing the development of pitting oedema. Transverse frictions may be used to encourage the development of mobile scar, and as a prelude to manipulation for scar tissue rupture in a chronic injury. Grade two and three injuries present with marked swelling and are protected non-weight bearing (severe injury) or preferably partial weight bearing with a compression bandage. Where minimal swelling indicates a grade one injury, an eversion strapping may be applied to protect the ligament from inversion stresses and to shorten it.

Rehabiliatation of the ankle aims to restore mobility, strength and function. For inversion, eversion, dorsiflexion and plantarflexion, together with combinations of these movements, resisted exercise using rubber powerbands may be used. Maximum repetitions are used to restore muscle endurance, while strength is developed using maximal resistance. With the band placed over both forefeet, eversionl movements may be performed. One end of the band is placed around a table leg and the other over the foot for performing the other movements.

Partial, and then full, weight bearing exercises may be used to develop strength in a closed kinetic chain position. In single leg standing with the support of wall, trunk movements are performed to throw stress onto the ankle, in addition exercises such as heel raising, toe lifts, and inversion and or eversion are performed. A balance beam (flamingo balance) is used, and again trunk and hip movements of the contralateral limb throw stress onto the injured ankle. The foot may be placed along the beam, or with the beam travelling transversely and only the toes supported. As the player attempts to maintain his or her balance on the balance bar, intense muscle activity is seen around the ankle. The stresses imposed on the various points of the feet may be altered by varying the player's footwear and performing the exercises in bare feet.

A balance board with a longitudinal rib is used for frontal plane actions and a single transverse rib is used for sagittal movements. A board with a domed central raise is used to combine movements for circumduction. Actions such as catching and throwing while standing on the balance board are helpful, in addition to trunk movements, as these actions take the player's attention away from the ankle. It will increase the skill of the player. Running, hopping and jumping activities may be used to develop power of the ankle. Running in a circle, figure-of-eight and on hills may change the stress on the ankle. All these activities may be done on varying surfaces like sand, gras etc.

SPECIFIC INJURIES

Fractures:

The most frequent ankle fracture is for instance, a deltoid ligament repture may avulse the medial malleolus and lead to a spiral fracture of the distal fibula. In the same way, rupture of the lateral collateral ligament can lead to a vertical fracture of the medial malleolus. These fractures must be associated with the lateral fracture. Similarly, tibiofibular ligament damage can be accompanied by a medial malleolus fracture due to eversion. Deltoid ligament injury may cause the distal tibiofibular fracture at the joint line. Transverse malleolar fractures are the result of avulsion injuries, whereas compression of the talus will result in vertical malleolar fractures. Displaced malleolar fractures are mostly coexisted by ligamentous injury. Compression forces that injure the ankle may also damage the spine and calcaneus.

Stable injuries due to a single fracture or ligament tear require no reduction and can be treated with a posterior splint and the RICE (Rest, Ice & Immobilization, Compression, and Elevation) regimen, followed by a walking for four to six weeks. Unstable injuries resulting from a sprain, a fracture, or various combination thereof, require reduction (Walsh & Hughston, 1976). Unstable injuries tend to have a very high incidence of complications, e.g. traumatic arthritis, persistent talar instability or ossification of the interosseus membranes.

Isometric exercises or early range of motion exercises in a hinge cast will minimize the harmful effects of immobilization i.e. stiffness and muscle atrophy.

Several studies suggested that small fragments of subchondral bone and overlying articular cartilage can be separated from the talar dome due to compressive or repetitive shearing type loads particularly in forced plantarflexion. Injurious change may be located anywhere on the talar dome. Gradual onset pain is also there which becomes worse over weeks or even months. This pain may increases with exercise and normally causes ankle stiffness or locking. After diagnosis of loose fragment in this area, orthopedic consultation should be considered.

Strains:

Ankle is always a subject of static and dynamic forces so

strains of ankle joint are very common in a variety of sports. Simple switching over from street shoes to sports shoes can cause a static strain of the tibial muscles because street shoes or normal shoes have a firm medial support and heel with a strong contour, and sports shoes have no heel, minimal support and weak contour. Medial strains involve the tibialis anterior, whereas the tibialis posterior is normally liable at its attachment to the tuberosity of the naviculus or liable under its medial side due to its dual roles in effecting inversion and plantar flexion, as well as supporting the foot arch. Tenderness will usually be felt at the medial border of the arch, with some spread under the arch and the back of the medial malleolus. The tendoachilles can be strained at its site of attachment to the calcaneus, along the tendon's course, or most frequently at the musculotendinous junction.

Mack (1982) observed that stronger forces; particularly in a push off, landing in forceful dorsiflexion or in a forceful drive as in racquet sports, basketball or board-jumping; can result in spontaneous rupture of the tendon. General complain of the player will be of a sensation of being accidently kicked or struck by a ball in the back of the calf. On examination, a slight limp with variable amounts of edema and tenderness on palpation may be noted. If the observation is made at the time of accident, without wasting anytime, a palpable gap will be noticed and if this will done after several hours swelling may conceal the gap. Active range of motion will still preserve plantar flexion due to imtact peroneal, tibial and toe flexor muscle groups.

Tibio-Talar Impingement Syndrome:

In the gymnastics and related games, repeated forced dorsiflexion may cause anterior impingement of the talus of the tibia. Pain occurs over the front of the ankle and is exacerbated by dorsiflexion with overpressure. Forced planterflexion in karate and football may cause posterior impingement giving pain over the back of the ankle without tenderness to the Achilles tendon.

In both the conditions, slight swelling and repeated impaction of the joint surfaces will be there which may lead to compression of the cartilage and subchondral bone. These structures do not show great sensitivity and will not be the primary source of pain. The existing pain come either from the periosteum, joint capsule, or more likely from chemical irritation and mechanical stress caused by the inflammatory response itself. Rest, anti-inflammatory modalities and training modification may give good results in this impingement syndromes.

Rapid, forceful dorsiflexion which may occur in a fall on to the feet, can force the talus up with enough force to stress the distal tibiofibular ligament. The joint is tender to palpation within the sulcus between the tibia and fibula, and pain is elicited to passive dorsiflexion. Strapping the foot to limit dorsiflexion and using a heel raise may be suggested as treatment.

Peronei:

One problem of ankle sprain is a strain or avulsion of the peroneus brevis where it attaches to the base of fifth metatarsal. According to McLennan (1980) and Stover (1980) the peroneal retinaculum can be torn with a direct blow to the back of the lateral malleolus while the tendons are taut in eversion and dorsiflexion. Peroneal tendon dislocation may occur if the tip of the lateral malleolus is fractured with forced dorsiflexion or a direct blow. As the foot is dorsiflexed, local pain is there and pain may reduce as the foot is plantarflexed.

Acute subluxation of the peroneal tendon is relatively uncommon and is most often confused with simple lateral ligament sprains. The tenderness and swelling, however, are centered behind the lateral malleolus and extended proximally over the tendons. They are absent over the anterolateral ankle capsule, where they would usually be found in a typical lateral sprain. One or both the peroneal tendons may pop out of the groove onto the lateral aspect of the malleolus. Reduction is usually spontaneous. Untreated acute episodes or congenital weakness will result in chronic or recurrent subluxation of the peroneal tendons.

CHAPTER-6

Injuries of Knee Joints

Majority of a cute knee injuries result from a valgus and/ or twisting strain. In majority of cases they involve the medial joint structures and the anterior cruciate ligament, which has a decisive role in the functional integrity of the tibiofemoral joint. The menisci and patellogemoral joint mechanism are also frequent sites of injury. The use of arthroscope is very helpful for diagnosis in acute knee injuries.

Applied Anatomy and Biomechanics :

In the body, patella is the largest sesamoid bone. This bone is attached above to the quadriceps tendon, below to the patellar tendon, and medially and laterally to the patellar retinacula. The breadth of the pelvis and close proximity of the knee creates a valgus angulation to the femur. Coupled with this, the direction of the pull of the quadriceps is along the shaft of the femur and that of the patellar tendon is almost vertical. The difference between the two lines of pull is known as the Q angle. This angle is an important determinant of knee health. Normal values for the Q angle are in the region of 15 to 20 degree. Knees with an angle greater or less than this angle can be considered malaligned.

The knee has cualities of flexion and extension, so the patella should move in line with the long axis of the femur. However, the horizontal force vector created as a result of the Q angle tends to pull the patella laterally, a movement which is resisted by the horizontal pull of the lower fibres of vastus medialis. According to Speakman and Weisberg (1977) these lower fibres can be considered as a functionally separate muscle viz. the vastus medialis oblique. The quadriceps as a whole have been shown to undergo reflex inhibition as the knees wells. Arno (1990) found that the vastus medialis oblique could be restrained by as little as 10 ml. effusion while the vastus lateralis and rectus femoris require as much as 60 ml. Minimal effusion occurs normally with minor trauma and the athlete may not be aware of this trauma. This effusion will be enough to weaken the vastus medialis oblique and change the biomechanics of the patella.

Patella does not contact the femur in his full extension position but lies in a lateral position. In the process of flexion, patella should move medially. If it moves laterally it will knock the prominent lateral femoral condyle, and the lateral edge of the patellar groove of the femur. As flexion progresses different areas of the patella's undersurface are compressed on to the femur. At 20 degree flexion the inferior pole of the patella is compressed and by 45 degree the middle section is affected. AT 90 degree flexion, compression has moved to the superior aspect of the knee. In a full squatting position, with the knee reaching 135 degree flexion, only the medial and lateral areas of the patella are compressed (Norris, 1993).

Cox (1990) opines that patello- femoral loads may be as high as three or four times body weight as the knee flexes in walking, and nine times body weight when descending stairs. The effect of the Q angle is to create both horizontal and vertical force vectors which tend to compress the lateral aspect of the patella but submit the medial aspect too tensile stress. While the posterior surface of the patella is compressed, the anterior aspect received a tensile force. Alterations in the Q angle will change the pattern of stress experienced by the patellar cartilage. Knee angles in the stance phase of walking or running will be altered by foot and hip mechanics through the closed kinetic chain.

Specific Injuries

Patellar Dislocation :

It is often an isolated injury and it may be associated with more extensive derangements of the knee joint. It may occur traumatically with any athlete but children between the age-group of 8-15 years and middle-aged women who are overweight and have poor muscular development of the quadriceps are more susceptible to this problem. Biomechanically, the individual is more susceptible to patellar dislocation if they demonstrate genu valgum, excessive femoral anteversion or external rotation of the tibia, and those who have weak vastus medialis oblique.

Normally patellar dislocation occur when the athlete for example turns to the left while pushing off from the right foot because the knee is externally rotated and straightened at the same time. This occurs because of the tibial attachment of the quadriceps move laterally in relation to the femur, increasing the lateral force component as the muscle group contracts. The patella almost always dislocated laterally. The patella dislocation is coexisted by a ripping sensation and excruciating pain, causing the knee to give way. Due to haemarthrosis, there is swelling in the injured knee. Normally, athlete is completely disabled by pain and quadriceps spasm.

Complete immobilization of the knee may be initial treatment of this dislocation. If pain is intense, aspiration may be required but usually swelling diminishes with non-invasive management. Only when 90 degree knee flexion is achieved and the patient is able to perform a straight leg lift with 30-50% of the power of the uninjured leg, may be allowed to walk without support. Without healing of medial ratina- culum, the athlete should not be allowed to mobilize with unprotected knee.

Patellar Fracture :

Usually, as a result of jumping, patellar fracture may occur. Most frequently, adolescent athletes are the victim of this injury. Fracture my occur at the pole of the patella. Jerosch, etl (1989) observed that stress fracture at the distal third of the patella has been reported after sprinting.

Mobility exercises and quadriceps strengthening may be used for the treatment of this fracture. Strengthening begins with straight leg raising Exler (1991) feels that immobilizing the limb in a cast for two to three weeks is sufficient in 50-60% of cases. The leg is locked from a long sitting position and, as it is raised, the tibia falls 2-3 cm. as the patient is unable to maintain locking. Patient may be re-educated the knee-locking mechanism through side-lying (gravity eliminated) position. Re-education of knee-locking mechanism may also be achieved by knee bracing with a rolled towel under the knee. The patient being instructed to push down on the towel with the back of the knee and at the same time to lift the heel from the couch surface.

Medial Collateral Ligament Injury :

It is a commonest injury to the knee resulting from the combination of valgus and extemal rotation force. There are three grades of medial collateral ligament injury :

Sprain of the Superficial Medial Collateral Ligament : In this injury there is sprain of the superficial medial collateral ligament but there is no demonstrable laxity or it is minimal. A full range of movement is found with discomfort only at the extreme of flexion. On stressing this ligament in 30 degree flexion there is discomfort, though no instability found in this injury. At the site of the sprain, usually the femoral attachment, tenderness and minimal soft tissue swelling are found. Anti-inflammatory modalities, resisted quadriceps contraction and early range of motion exercise may be used for treatment of this injury. Immobilization which restricts knee flexion, is prohibited.

Partial Tear of the Superficial Medial Collateral Ligament :Laxity may be demonstrated in this injury though the deep layer is intact. Initially, the extension is uncomfortable and the knee is stable tot valgus stress in extension. There is a small swelling, approximately the size of a half walnut, usually at the femoral attachment. Tenderness is localized to the tear.

Combination of early mobilization and functional support for acute ligamentous instability are backbone of the therapy. If mobilization is allowed to take place without functional support there is risk of the development of ectopic calcification at the site of the injury. An ambulatory cast brace may be used to control the rotational movement at the knee. This should be maintained for three weeks and then the cast brace should be removed. After removal of the cast brace, patient may be referred for flexibility, strengthening and proprioceptive exercises.

In a less severe injury, crutches may be used for several days. At that time variety of motion exercises are also instituted. Within a week patients may have regained the full range of motion and then a cycling program may be started. A progressive rehabilitation programme is continued until full power and endurance have been regained. .

Complete Tear of Medial Collateral Ligament : It is a grade III injury in which tear involves both superficial and deep layers of ligaments. It may be an isolated injury, although normally it is associated with medial meniscus tear, anterior cruciate ligament tear or patella dislocation. Due to this injury there is a significant functional disturbance. Bleeding and oedema cause diffuse swelling. Additional features which suggests a complete tear are an empty feeling i.e. a mushy end-point on performing the valgus stress test in 30 degree flexion.

Tears of Anterior Cruciate Ligaments :

These injuries are most problematic. Amount of ligament tissue torn, location of tear, associated meniscal damage, congenital laxity of the joints, and the athlete's functional goals are the factors which predict this injury. All the anterior cruciate ligament injuries should be referred to an orthopedic surgeon. After determining the amount of intra-articular damage, a treatment programme can be formulated. Damaged menisci may require repair or removal. If the injury to the cruciate ligament is only partial, and laxity is mild, the patient may not require surgical repair. Usually the tear occurs in the middle third of the ligament, so that the cruciate's tenuous blood supply is disrupted and no direct repair is possible. In this instance, an immediate augmentation or substitution type of procedure may be chosen.

Prosterior Cruciate Ligament Tears :

This ligament has a most important stabilizing function. Baylis and Rzonca (1988) found that this ligament is the strongest ligament in the knee. Its basic restraining function is to check posterior displacement of the tibia. When the ligament is ruptured, symptoms are often sufficiently disabling to prevent involvement in body contact sports.

Immediate pain is felt by the athlete and he may experience difficulty in weight bearing. On the site of injury there may be swelling which is dependent upon the extent of injury.

Symptoms of posterior cruciate tear are as follows :

1. If the patient lyes on back with face upwards, hip flexed to 45 degree and knee flexed to 90 degree; the tibia drops back on the femur. It is called posterior sag sign. If both the hip and knee are flexed to 90 and the heel is supported by the

physician, the sag may be seen.

2. When posterior stress is applied during rotation with the hip flexed to 45 degree, and the knee flexed to 90 degree posterorotatory subluxation of the respective tibial plateaux may be found.
3. When the legs are held by the toes and lifted off the couch, the affected knee slips back into hyperextension and the tibia rotates laterally. A positive result of external rotation/ recurvatum test indicates posterolateral instability.

The knee with only posterior cruciate ligament damage producing unidirectional instability generally does well conservatively but when this damage is associated with additional tissue damage which results in multidirectional instability, surgery should be considered (Torg, 1989).

Haemarthrosis :

Initial task of the physician is to distinguish between haemarthrosis and serious joint effusion because of similarity of symptoms in both the injuries. The initial clue lies in the history: swelling that occurs within an hour or two of injury, giving rise to a feeling of joint tightness, is most likely due to bleeding - that is, a haemarthrosis. However a joint effusion develops overnight. It is noticed by the patient in the next morning after injury. Another difference lies in the size of joint swelling. A haemarthrosis is a tense joint containing upto 100 ml. of blood. A serious effusion associated with osteochondritis dissecans or a torn meniscus, without chronic or recurring rheumatological problem, results in a much smaller swelling.

Haemarthrosis of knee due to acute injury, the likely diagnosis are rupture of the anterior cruciate ligament, peripheral meniscus tear or patella dislocation. Noyexs etl (1980) found that anterior cruciate ligament rupture occurred in 72% of cases of traumatic haemarthrosis without significant collateral ligament injury on clinical examination.

Management strategies are dependent upon establishment of the underlying cause of the haemarthrosis. Aspiration may be performed for confirmation of the haemarthrosis and/or for comfort of patient.

Meniscal Injury :

The menisci rest on the tibial condyles. When viewed from above, they seem like crescent but triangular in cross-section. Peripheral border of menisci is formed from fibrous tissue and attached to the deep surface of the joint capsule. These same fibres attach the menisci to the tibial surface forming the coronary ligaments. According to Palastanga, Field, and Soames (1989) anteriorly, the two menisci are joined by the transverse ligament and posterior transverse ligament being present in 20% of the population.

The medial meniscus is the larger between the two. Its shape is semicircular. Anterior horn of the medial meniscus is attached to the front of intercondylar area of the tibia in front of the anterior cruciate ligament. Its posterior horn attache to the posterior intercondylar area between the posterior cruciate ligament and the lateral meniscus. It has an attachment to the oblique popliteal ligament coming from semimembranosus and the medial collateral legament. The upper part of the meniscus is firmly attached to this ligament. The fibres here forming the medial meniscus-femoral ligament. The lower part of the meniscus which is more lax, attached to the coronary ligament.

Shape of lateral meniscus is more circular and has a uniform breadth. Two horns of lateral meniscus are closely attached with each other. The anterior horn blending with the attachment of the anterior cruciate ligament. The posterior horn attaches just anterior to the posterior horn of the medial meniscus.

Kelley (1990) estimated that meniscal injury occur with a frequency of 61 per one lakh population. Males are three times more vulnerable than females and medial meniscal injury is four times more prevalent than lateral meniscal injury.

History of meniscal injury is normally one which combines twisting on a semiflexed knee with the foot fixed on the ground. Starting of this problem is sudden and pain is felt deep within the knee. Effusion may be extensive after injury, and haemarthrosis may result if the injury occurs with the damage of anterior cruciate ligament or medial collateral legament. Effusion is apparent and tenderness is often found over the joint line. A capsular pattern may be noticeable, like gross limitation of flexion and slight limitation of extension. Terminal extension is often blocked with a springy end feel if muscle spasm is not present. Various tests are used to assess the problem.

Henning (1988) recommended that meniscal tears of less than 10 mm in length and partial thickness injuries involving 50% or less of the vertical height of the meniscus could be treated non-operatively, if anterior cruciate ligament was undamaged. Weiss etl (1989) found that stable vertical longitudinal tears in the vascular outer area of the meniscus had a good potential for healing but stable radial tears did not have this power.

CHAPTER-7

Prevention of Sports Injury

The term 'prevention' is normally used in the context of sports injuries refers to any measure which can stop an injury occurring. Process of prevention also play an important role to minimize the injury and ensure that the same injury does not recur.

There are so many causes of sports injuries. Failure in technique, faulty sports equipment, poor physical fitness, inadequate warm-up and psychological factors were identified as the causes of sports injuries by Williams and Sperryn (1976). Taimela, Kujala and Osterman (1990) divided injury risk factors into intrinsic and extrinsic groups. Intrinsic factors are age, gender, Somato type, local anatomy and biomechanics, fitness, physical symmetry, joint integrity, motor control, and psychological or psychosocial factors. Extrinsic factors of sports injuries are organization and management, type of sport, training errors environment and equipment. Aim of the coach should be to reduce these risk factors to a minimum.

Protective Equipment:

Use of protective equipment in various sports results as the reduction in the incidence of sports injury. Now in almost every recognized tournaments wearing of these equipments of acceptable design is mandatory. Use of these equipments in a proper way is also essential. An obvious example is the wearing of suitable helmets. Even when a helmet is worn, it is important to stress the need for attachment of the chinstrip. Fashion plays an important role in the development of various protective equipments. Not long age, Mike Brearley (an outstanding captain of English cricket) was advocating the use of head and facial protection while batting at cricket. At first, the reaction from other side was of disbelief, but the application of protection in specific risk situations, for example batting or fielding close to the wicket, is now a common feature. In some sports e.g. cricket, hockey and motorcycling, the helmet has a visor or grille extension to reduce the incidence of maxillofacial injury. In cricket batsmen often protect the forearms and thighs as well as genitals. In karate the use of fist pads has been shown to reduce the severity of head injuries, which account for the ma ority of injuries sustained in tournaments.

Goggles are worn in a number of sports in which high speeds are encountered. Special goggles made from tough polycarbonate material for many sports. General public is interested to replace spectacles by contact lens but in sports one should not assume that the mere replacement of spectacles by contact lenses protects the eye. Increased damage to the eye may result from direct trauma to a contact lens. Soft lenses are sofest.

In almost all the sports, shoes are used by the participants. There has been a considerable improvement in design of sports shoes over the last decade. An unsatisfactory level of support or shock absorption may be associated with inadequate heel counter, inadequate arch support, disruption between the upper and the sole, and/or early deterioration of the shock-absorbing properties of the midsole. Pressure effects which give rise to brusitis or tendinitis, may be due to the laces that are too tight, insufficient breadth of shoe, irritation from the heel tab, anatomical foot deformities and/or biomechanical abnormalities.

All contact sports participants are at risk. The highest incidence of injury to mouth and teeth are in boxing. So the mouth guards are compulsory for boxing. Non-contact sports like hockey and football, are not exempted from these direct trauma. Use of mouth guards in the sports is encouraged though not mandatory. A suitable protector acts against trauma to the teeth and lips. On the other hand, the likelihood of laceration of lips, mouth and tongue from the teeth is drastically reduced. A variety of mouth guards are available. An inexpensive guard made from the thermoplastic material and moulded by the user usually fits better though it may not be sufficiently extensive or resilient at points of maximal stress. Second type of guard viz. 'off the shelf' are the least adequate. They may fit badly and easily be displaced. A custom made mouth guard constructed from a cast impression taken by a dental surgeon is the most satisfactory.

Specific type of clothing is important in certain sports. Fireproof materials are useful in the clothes of racing drivers. Light-weight emergency anti-explosure clothing should be carried by mountaineers to protect against sudden changes in the weather.

Environment :

The field of play should be the focus of attention, especially in amateur sports. It is the main responsibility of coach to inspect the field before starting the game. In gymnastics the basic basement requirement of 1½ inches of padding should be augmented by mats of 4 inch thickness around the various pieces of equipment. Indoor are as should be designed to exclude obstacles such as radiator, which are potential sources of injury.

Another aspect of environment that warrants attention is the other players. In youth sports, players should be matched for size and maturity. Where the age-group of players covers a wide range, there may be a great difference in body size due to the premature development of some youngsters. Especially in contact sports a 14-year old athlete who is 1.6m.. tall and weighs 75kgs. should not be given permission to play opposite a 10-year old who is 1.3m tall and weights 46 kgs.

Screening :

The subject of physical screening of youngsters in sport is one which attracts much discussion. A variety of anatomical abnormalities may develop largely unnoticed to the lay man. However, these can often be readily identified by the sports medicine practitioner with a series of annual screening tests.

Guidelines on individuals fitness to compete should be framed in consultation with the important and relevant sports bodies. This practice of medical screening may vary from country to country. These guidelines may prevent sports person from variety of illness and injuries. For instance, the existence of hyperextension of the knees or hypermobility in general have a risk of ligament and/or joint injury.

Participation in certain sports or recreational activities like swimming requires a medical examination. Some sports require medical certification, if the participant has reached a certain age, for example parachuting requires this certificate for the participant of above 40 years of age.

Physiological components which may contribute to athletic performance may be outlined as under:

Physique **:** In sports like football it is quite clear that size of players is as important as their explosive power. On the other hand, variation in body size of 800 m. runners is quite comprehensive. The determination of body fat per unit body weight is of more relevance and may be calculated by the use of skin-clippers. Alternatively, lean body weight may be determined by electrical impedance.

Flexibility : The measurement of flexibility should not be confined to an isolated test for combined trunk flexion and hamstring elasticity, despite its relative importance. All the major joints are examined. At very mobile joints range of motion in the position of function is recorded. External rotation in 90 degree abduction of the shoulder is essential for tennis players. Hyperemobility should be recorded if present. Although at first sight, this would appear to be beneficial in, e.g. gymnastics and dance, there is an increased incidence of injury and osteoarthrosis in later life (SCOTTETAL, 1979).

Muscle strength and power : Though strength plays an important role in a number of sports but due to the lack of inherent definition it is measured in a number of ways. Some are using sophisticated apparatus to measure this strength and some are making crude judgment through field test.

Hutson (1996) suggests to use the lido isokinetic dynamometer for this purpose due to following reasons:

1. determination of fatigue index- an anaerobic test of local muscle endurance,
2. establishment of data base of muscle function for fit individuals or team members,
3. detection of muscle inbalance as an assessment procedure

or in established injury, for example, comparison of torque ratios of a agonists and antagonists,

4. rehabilitation after injury, and
5. isokinetic training.

Technique :

Due to inadequate technique there are abnormal biomechanical strains upon the athlete's musculoskeletal system. Vigilance is required by the trainers in order to prevent injury from poor technique. If the trainer is vigilant regarding the postures in certain exercises, the incidence of low back problems including spondylolysis, in young dancers should be kept minimum. Care should be taken to avoid an excessive lordosis at the barre and in floor exercises. Correct lifting technique is useful to reduce lordotic stress in older male dancers. Excessive pelvic flexion or extension will increase the likelihood of injury.

If technique is faulty, the pivotal area of the spine is at risk. Too much forward swing prior to powerful leg action in rowers should be prohibited. Hyperextension and hyperflexion, in air as well as on water entry is a cause of low back injury in highboard divers. For swimmers low back pain is a result of overuse of the butterfly stroke.

In field athletics also this technique is important. For example, in javelin throwing power is maximized by rotation of the body and chest. During the throw, the knee ipsilateral to the throwing arm is brought through quickly to block forward momentum and 'square off' the body, thereby reducing the likelihood of a side-arm throw, which is more likely to incur shoulder strain.

Psychological Factors :

Psychological factors have a significant effect on an athlete's capacity for training and motivation for competition. Athletes of a certain psychological type may be more predisposed to injury. Sports coach most recognize these characteristics. Factors which are generally believed to influence sports performance include aggression, motivation, anxiety, concentration, self-confidence, emotional state and pain tolerance. With the help of sports psychologists personality profile of each player may be prepared which may help the trainers in training camps.

Knowledge of Sports Mechanism :

Basic knowledge of sports mechanics is essential to appreciate the factors which is involved in prevention of injury as well as management of injury. Attention should be given to such concepts as force, force around an axis of rotation (torque), centre of gravity etc. Torque itself has great relevance in certain joints like subtalar joint. In other joints the resultant force in different positions of the surrounding levers is of great relevance- e.g. in the patellofemoral joint. Muscle function depends on its physiological state of training. The ground reactive factors i.e. those forces which are applied to the body by contact with the ground, depend on the magnitude of the force with which the athlete presses on the ground. Nigg (1988) stated that such external vertical forces amount to two and a half to three times the body weight in running and may increase to three or four times the body weight in jumping. The suitability of shock absorption, either in the training shoe or the training surface, is an important consideration in he prevention of these injuries.

In sprinting, high knee action is coupled with early elevation of the heel toward the buttock as soon as the foot leaves the ground rapid leg movement is achieved by the use of a small swing radius. So, the training should concentrate on strengthening these muscle and creating a balance with the gluteals and the quadriceps. Running style of long distance runners, in comparison to sprinters, is quite different. Here muscle economy is required. Although powerful hamstrings are not required, nevertheless the athlete is at risk of developing hamstring contrature unless flexibility exercises are performed regularly.

Warm up :

Warm-up may be either passive or active. In passive warm-up external heat source is used and in active warm-up body heat is used.

The effects of warm-up seem to be physiological, psychological and biomechanical. Physiological effects are largely due to increases in tissue temperature, while psychological effects are mainly due to practice. Biomechanical effects are achieved by alterations in the tissue response to mechanical strain.

A general warm-up, intense enough to induce mild sweating without causing fatigue,is important for injury prevention. The general activity should be followed by a specific warm-up designed to produce a suitable arousal level in the athlete, and to rehearse any complex skills which will be used later in competitions.

In vigorous exercise; joints, muscle and other soft tissues should be extended through their full physiological range before competition. During this phase intensity should be tailored, depending upon the baseline of fitness, to increase aerobic capacity.

It is also important that the vigorous exercise does not end abruptly, but slows gradually during a cool down period. During this phase body metabolism is allowed to return to normal gradually by the inclusion of a reduced level of muscle activity.

CHAPTER-8

FIRST AID

What is First Aid?

First aid is the immediate care given to an injured or sick person until the services of a physician can be obtained.

Value of Having First Aid Knowledge

If you know how to give first aid properly, you are able to help others when they need help most. When someone is injured, people are always willing to help. But often, because the have not studied first aid, they make mistakes and injure the victim even more. The good first aider know what to do and also what not to do.

By giving proper care you may save lives or prevent lifelong crippling. You will decrease suffering and perhaps cause the accident or illness expenses to be less than they otherwise would be. Many young people have become heroes because they knew what to do in case of drowning, injuries, bleeding and so on. Another important result of studying about accidents is that you become more careful and have fewer accidents or yourself. In addition, if you are injured you may be able to give yourself good first aid or to direct others to do so properly for you.

What is Shock?

When a person is badly injured, he may develop a serious condition called shock. In shock cases, the blood flow in the body is disturbed, even in parts distant from the injury. The brain does not get enough blood. Thinking is difficult, digestion of food is slowed, and all body processes are at a low level. The injured person feels exceedingly weak. Unless he receives proper care, he may die of shock, or his recovery may be greatly delayed.

Causes of Shock

Any serious injury may cause shock. Bad burns, loss of much blood, broken bones, and large cuts are often followed by shock. During World War II millions of Americans gave blood through the Red Cross for use by doctors in treating hock resulting from war wounds. At present there are many centers operated by the Red Cross and other organizations where people can contribute blood.

Signs of Shock

The skin of a person in shock feels cool and is whiter than usual. Sometimes perspiration appears, especially on the forehead or chin, or above the mouth. Sometimes the victim feels like vomiting or actually dies vomit.

First Aid of Shock

Whenever you give first aid to a seriously injured person, always try to prevent shock. Act immediately. Do not wait for shock to appear.

Make the victim lie down at one, so that his head is level with or lower than the rest of his body. However, if his breathing in this position is difficult because of chest injuries, raise the head and shoulders by placing pillows under them.

Cover him properly. Carefully place a blanket under him. If weather is not hot, place a coat or blanket over him. If the weather is very cool, use several blankets. But don't make him sweat; too much covering is undesirable.

Ordinarily you should not use hot water bottles or electric heating pads on accident victim. However, you may use them if the weather is very cold and there aren't enough blankets. The best places to use them are under the armpits or about the chest. To prevent burning the skin, they should be only slightly warmer than body temperature.

Give warm water to drink if an hour or more will pass before the doctor sees the victim. But if the doctor will see him soon, give nothing to drink. In any case, don't give water if the person is unconscicus or has an injury in the stomach region. Stimulants such as ammonia have no value in shock.

Don't disturb the injured person unnecessarily. Try to avoid measures that would cause more pain. Unnecessary handling and careless transportation make shock worse.. It is best not to question the victim much or to discuss his injuries. Don't feed him. He should lie as quiet as possible.

These first aid measure-having the victim lie flat and providing the proper amount of covering-are very important. They help prevent shock; therefore, apply them at once. They also help if shock does develop.

WOUNDS; DRESSINGS AND BANDAGES

WOUNDS

A wound is an injury in which the skin is cut or penetrated. For instance, a knife, bullet, ice pick, or wood splinter may inflict a wound. If the wound is deep, severe bleeding may occur, or there may be serious damage to structures within the body, such as the stomach, lungs, or brain.

In all wounds, even in small cuts or tiny stab wounds, there is danger that germs will grow in the wound, causing an infection.

What are Germs?

Germs are tiny living things, so small that they cannot be seen except with a microscope. Many germs are helpful to man, but some cause harm. They are everywhere about us, in the soil and water, in our homes, on our clothes and bodies, and even in our mouths and noes. The skin is a strong protect against harmful germs, because germ usually cannot work their way through the skin unless it is damaged.

What is Infection?

Whenever we suffer a cut, germs are sure to enter the wound, being carried in with the object that cuts, us or being pushed in from our clothes or skin. If the germs grow in the wound and harm us, an infection of the wound is present.

The signs of a wound infection are these: The skin become red and tender around the wound, some swelling may occur, and sometimes pus forms. These signs usually appear several day after the wound is received, though sometimes they occur within a shorter or a much longer time.

First Aid for Wounds in Which Bleeding Is Not Severe

The first aider should prevent more germs from entering the wound. Do not touch the wound or the skin near it with your fingers, with clothing, or with any other object. Do not breathe directly over the wound.

1. Apply over the wound a gauze dressing that is sterile-free from germs. Gauze dressings wrapped from paper and made sterile by heating can be purchased in drugstores. You must be careful when removing a dressing from its paper covering; wash your hands first and touch only a corner of the dressing when you apply it to the wound.
2. Apply a bandage over the dressing. This protect the wound still more and holds the dressing in place.
3. Send the victim to a doctor.

Sometimes sterile dressings are not at hand. In that case a clean cloth may be used. Many of the germs on the cloth can be killed by scorching it with a flame or hot iron or by washing the cloth in clean water-or better yet, in soap and water-and then drying it. Sometimes, as on a hike, even these measures may not be possible. If so, the first aider can expose the cloth to the direct rays of the sun for at least 10 minutes. When a cloth is applied to the wound it should be folded to make several layers.

Every wound, even though it is the tiniest scratch, should be properly cared for, lest a dangerous infection develop. Sometimes, when the wound is very small, people do not go to a doctor but try to treat it themselves. There are several ways to treat a tiny wound. The family doctor can tell you what to do. Perhaps he will advise that an antiseptic of his choice be applied carefully to the wound and to the skin around it. Antiseptic are preparations that kill germ. They also injure the body tissue somewhat. An increasing number of physicians advise that if people insist upon treating tiny wound themselves, they should apply no antiseptic, but should wash the wound thoroughly in boiled or clean water, permitting no dirt to remain. A sterile dressing and bandage should be placed upon a wound after first aid. People sometimes apply lard, butter, oils, or even tobacco juice to wounds. Such materials should not be used. Do not put adhesive tape directly on a wound and do not use cotton as a dressing.

It is much better to go to a doctor than to treat wounds yourself, even if they seem unimportant. Many people have paid dearly in money and illness because they tried to save money by treating injuries that seemed slight.

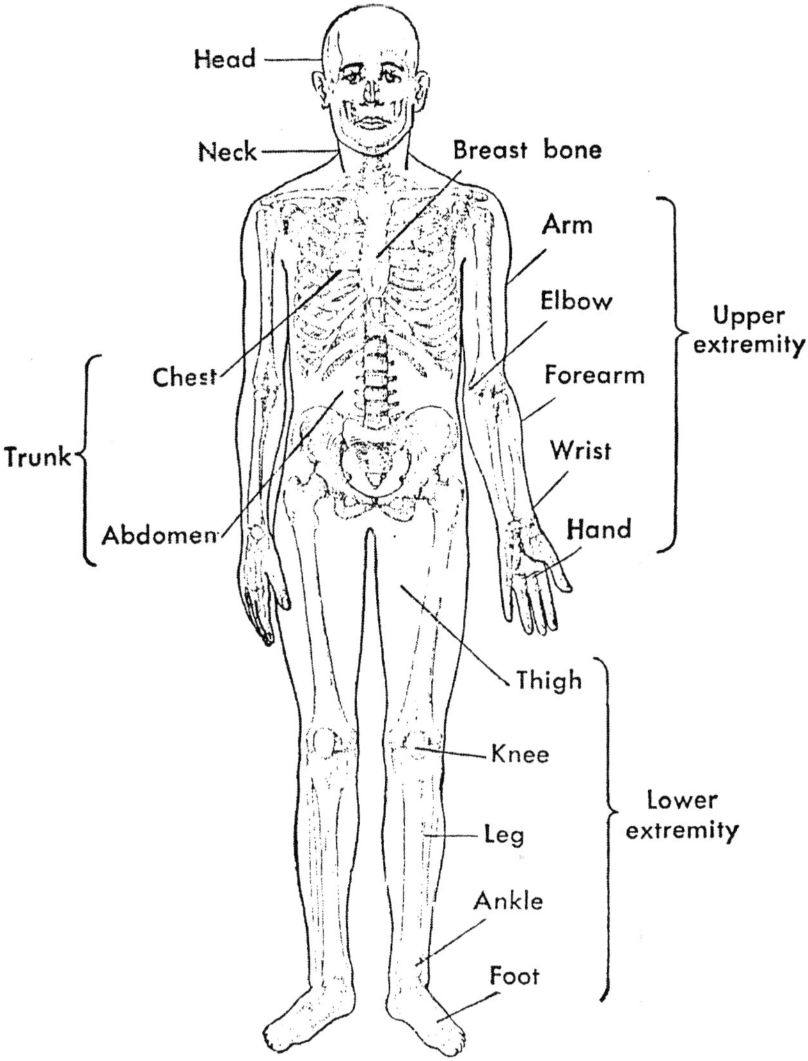

FIRST AID FOR BLEEDING

GENERAL FIRST AID MEASURES

Loss of a quart of blood by an adult or a proportionately smaller amount by a child is serious. This amount of blood can be lost within less than a minute if a large blood vessel is cut.

Therefore, serious bleeding should be stopped at once. You do not have time to call a doctor first. You must give this lifesaving first aid yourself without wasting a second of time.

In most cases you can stop bleeding by putting pressure directly on the bleeding part. It would be best if you thrust a sterile. Therefore you must apply pressure wit clothing or cloth at hand. This cloth should be folded to form a pad. Do not remove it, let bleeding recommence. If blood reddens the dressing, more dressing should be added.

Keep the bleeding person quiet. Do not excite him, or handle him roughly, or transport him carelessly, or talk to him unnecessarily.

If he will not soon be seen by a doctor, give him water, preferably warm, unless he is unconscious or has an injury in the stomach region. Treat him for shock and do not give him spirits or ammonia or other stimulants.

If a limb (extremity) is bleeding, raise it slightly above the rest of the body by placing blankets or some other object under the limb.

For severe bleeding of the upper or lower extremities two other measures are sometimes helpful-namely, the use of the tourniquet and the use of finger pressure.

Use of Tourniquet

A tourniquet (toor'-ni-ket) is a strip of cloth, rubber, or similar soft material that is wrapped tightly around the limb. Tourniquets should not be used if direct pressure will stop the bleeding-they may be harmful. A triangular bandage folded into a necktie shape make a good tourniquet. The band should be about 2 inches wide. A necktie, belt, or stocking can be used if better material is not available. Ropes, strings, wire, and very narrow strips of cloth do not make good tourniquets because they cut into the flesh and are painful.

The use of a tourniquet is seldom required. If it must be used, place the tourniquet close to the wound, but not at the wound edge. There should be unbroken skin between the tourniquet and the wound. Remember, it is always placed between the heart and the wound, never below the wound. Make sure it is applied tightly enough to stop bleeding. Once the tourniquet is applied, it should not be released, no matter how long it has been in place, except by a doctor. The doctor can control the bleeding properly and replace the blood the person has lost by blood transfusions. When a tourniquet is used, always make a note telling when and where it was applied. Tie the note to the victim where it can be seen. Tourniquet are applied only to the arms and legs and cannot be used for bleeding of the face, head, neck, or trunk of the body.

Use of Pressure Points

Use of finger pressure at pressure points is often helpful in case of bleeding from an extremity. It takes time to obtain material for a tourniquet and to apply it. If bleeding from the upper limb is extreme, you can apply finger pressure on the inner side of the arm. For bleeding in a lower extremity, apply the pressure at the point shown. Apply the pressure in these places even though the wound is in the lower part of extremity. By applying this finger pressure, you prevent blood from gong through the main vessel against the bone. Finger pressure in this way will not completely stop the bleeding but it will decrease it while you are getting a tourniquet ready, or while you apply a dressing firmly to the wound.

First Aid for Nosebleed

1. Sit up, holding the head tilted back very slightly.
2. Press the nostrils together, holding the pressure for several minute.
3. Apply a large towel, wet with cold water, over the nose and face.
4. Do not talk, cough, laugh, walk about, or blow the nose. Activity and excitement may increase the bleeding or cause it to restart.

THE BREATHING SYSTEM: ARTIFICIAL RESPIRATION

The process of breathing air in and out is called respiration. If a person's breathing is stopped by an accident, the first aider may give him artificial respiration; that is, he causes air to

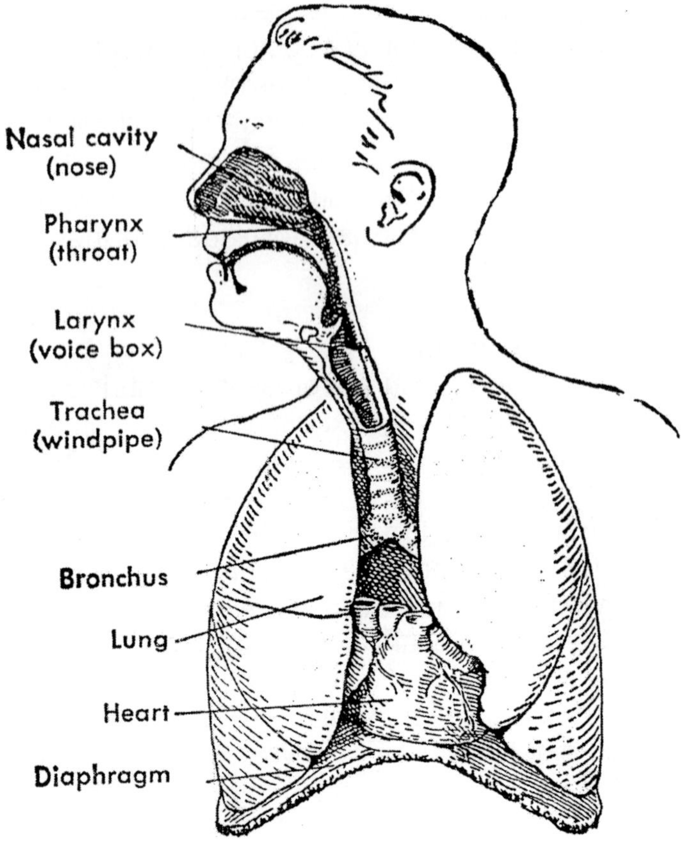

enter and leave the victim's lungs. A child can give artificial respiration just as well as an adult can. Giving artificial respiration to certain accident victims saves their lives.

Why Breathing Is Necessary

Oxygen, which is a part of the air, and food are carried by the blood to the body cells. There the food and oxygen unite, providing energy for our activities and heat to keep our bodies warm. The body quickly dies if it does not receive oxygen.

When food and oxygen unite, one product formed is a gas called carbon dioxide. Carbon dioxide has various uses, but because it is constantly forming, much of it must be thrown off. It is carried to the lungs and is expelled with the air we breathe out.

The Breathing Process

Air enters the nose and passes through the throat, windpipe, and bronchial tubes to the lungs. In the lungs the oxygen passes in to the blood capillaries.

When at rest, adults breathe about 1 times a minute, children somewhat faster. About a pint half quart of air is taken in and expelled during an average breath. You can take in much more air than this in a deep breath.

Take a deep breath. Observe that certain muscles in the chest wall cause the chest to increase in size. Meanwhile, a muscle (the diaphragm) at the base of the chest presses down against the abdominal cavity. As a result the chest cavity becomes larger and air rushes into the lungs. Then the muscles cease their efforts, the chest cavity becomes smaller, and air is expelled.

The Way To Give Artificial Respiration

The Red Cross teaches the back pressure-arm lift method.

1. Place the victim in a prone (face down) position with his hands under his head. Turn the face slightly to one side.
2. Kneel on one or both knee near the victim's head, facing his feet. Place your hands on his back so that the heels of your hands are just below and imaginary line running between the armpits and so that your thumbs just touch.
3. Rock forward slowly with elbow straight until your arms are approximately vertical, letting your weight gradually bear upon the victim. (In practice sessions, however, use only light pressure, especially if the pretended victim is smaller than you are.)
4. Immediately slide your hands to the victim's arms and rock slowly backward. As you rock, draw his arms upward and toward you until you feel definite tension at his shoulders. In this way you relieve the chest of some of the body weight. You need not raise his chest entirely off the floor. Repeat the cycle 12 times per minute, giving equal time to the press and the lift phases.

By pressing on the victim's chest in this way, you drive out some of the air from his body; when you lift his arms, air enters his

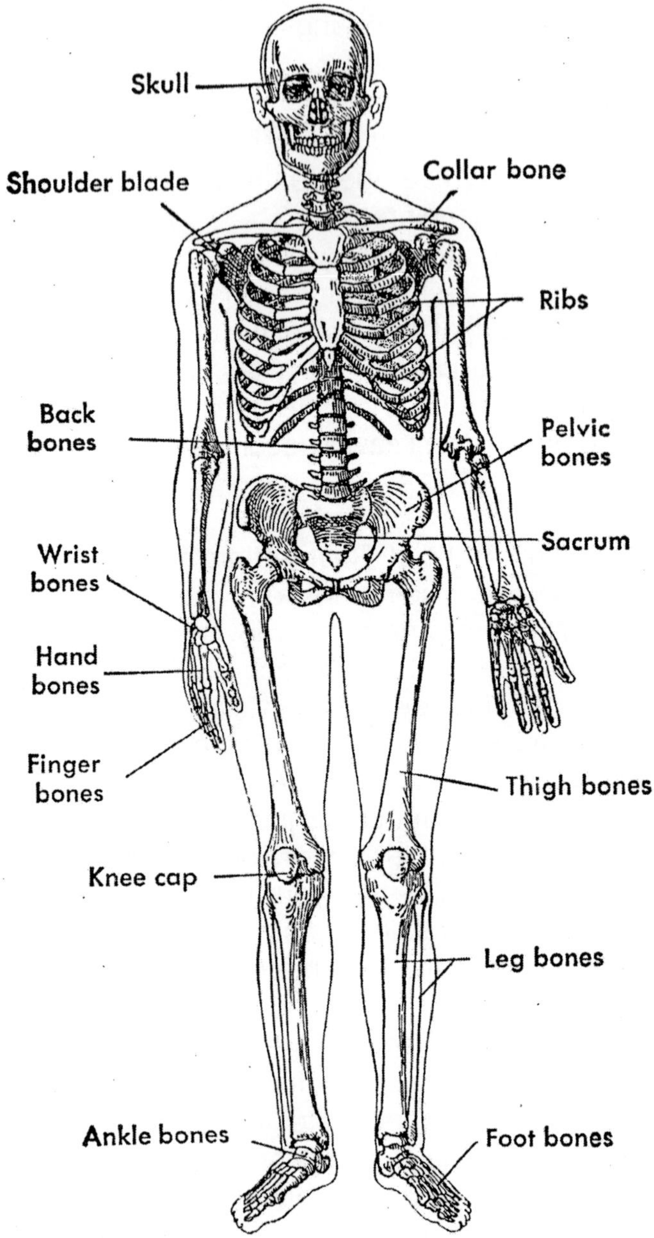
Skull
Shoulder blade
Collar bone
Ribs
Back bones
Pelvic bones
Sacrum
Wrist bones
Hand bones
Finger bones
Thigh bones
Knee cap
Leg bones
Ankle bones
Foot bones

body. The double movement of swinging forward and back should take about 5 seconds; therefore, the movements are repeated 12 times every minute.

Continue artificial respiration until the victim again breathes regularly of his own accord, or until the doctor comes and takes charge, or until you are positive that the victim is dead. The victim may start to breathe in less than 15 minute. In some cases, especially after electrical shock, several hours of artificial respiration may be necessary. It is easy to tell when the victim starts to breathe. You can feel breathing movements and sometimes you can hear gasping sounds. Continue artificial respiration until the breathing is regular. Then watch the victim and be ready to start again, because he may stop breathing.

There are other important first aid measure. Have someone call a doctor or ambulance at one. Have someone put blankets under and over the victim while you are giving artificial respiration. The necktie and collar should be loosened, and someone should pull slightly for a moment of the tip of the tongue to be sure that it is in place. After the victim recovers consciousness, he should not be allowed to get up until the doctor permits.

BODY FRAMEWORK; FRACTURES

Broken bones are common injuries. By giving good first aid to a person who has a broken bone, you may lessen disability and expense, or perhaps even save his life.

SKELETON (BODY FRAMEWORK)

There are over 200 bone in the human body. These bones form the framework or skeleton of the body.

The Skull

The bony part of the head is called the skull. The skull consists of 22 bones. In adulthood these bones, with one exception, have grown tightly together. The exception is the lower jaw. The upper and back part of the skull encloses the brain. The lower front part forms the framework for the face.

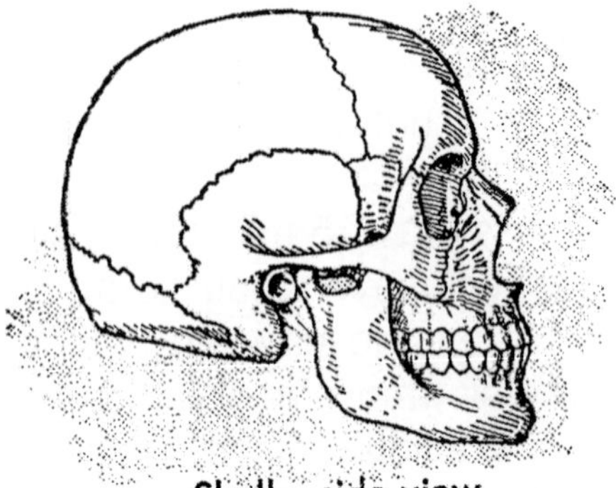

Skull—side view

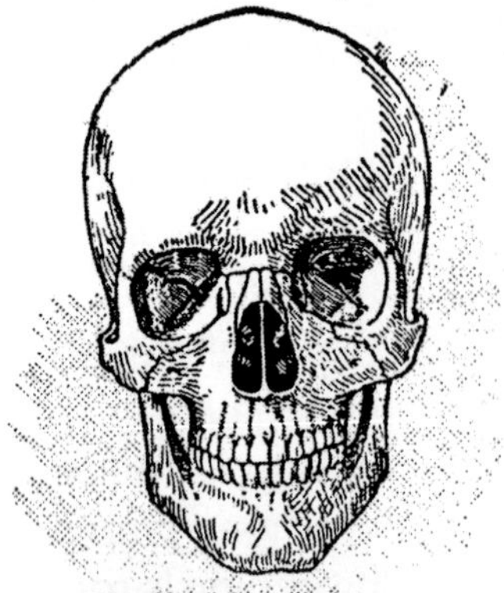

Skull—front view

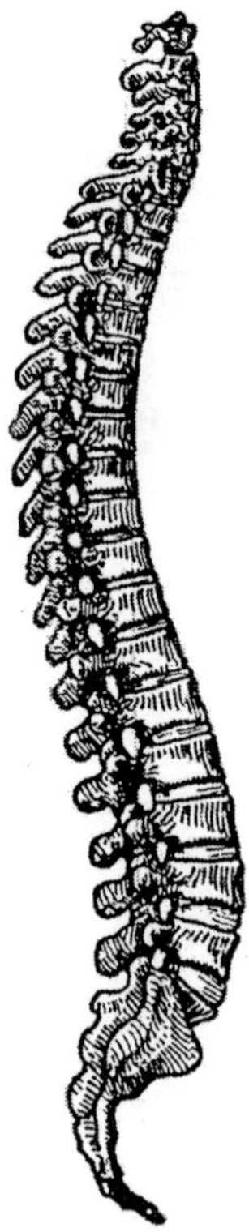

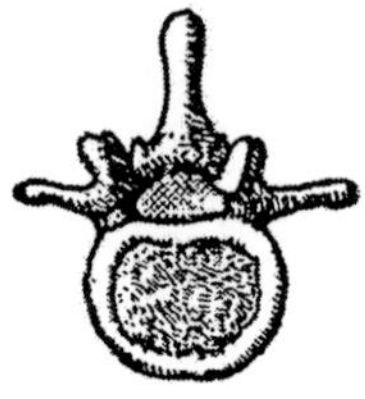

A vertebra

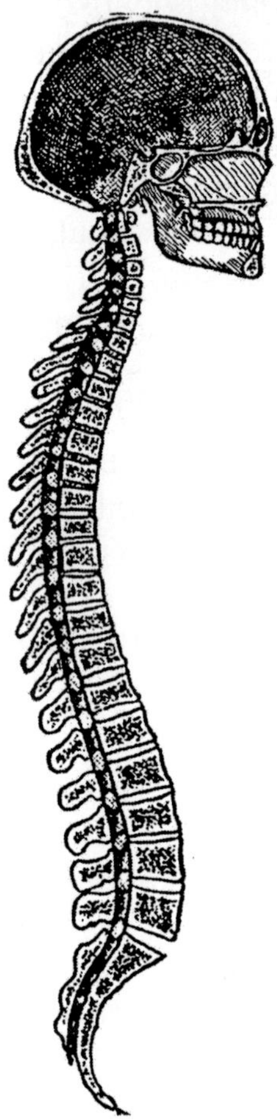

Spinal column

The Spinal Column

The skull rests on top of the spinal column (backbone or spine). The spinal column consists of many separate bones. Within each separate bones is a hole. The spinal cord, a large nerve passing downward from the brain, is contained within the holes in the backbone.

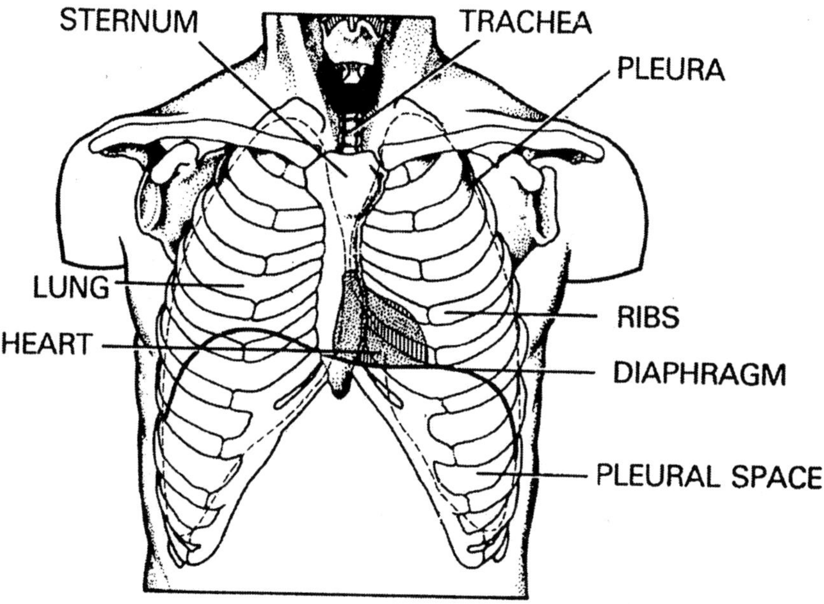

The Chest

There are 12 ribs on each side of the chest. They are attached in back to the spinal column. Most of them are attached to the breast bone in front, but the lower two on each side are not.

At the upper part of the chest are the two collarbones in front and the 2 shoulder blades in back. The arm bone fits into a socket in the shoulders blade.

The Pelvis

In the lower part of the trunk a ring of bones forms the pelvis.

The Upper Extremities

The upper extremity has one bone above the elbow, two in the forearm, eight in the wrist, and five in the palm. Each finger has three bones, but the thumb has only two.

The Lower Extremities

In the lower extremity there are one bone above the knee, two in the leg, and many in the feet. The kneecap is a bone located in front of the knee joint.

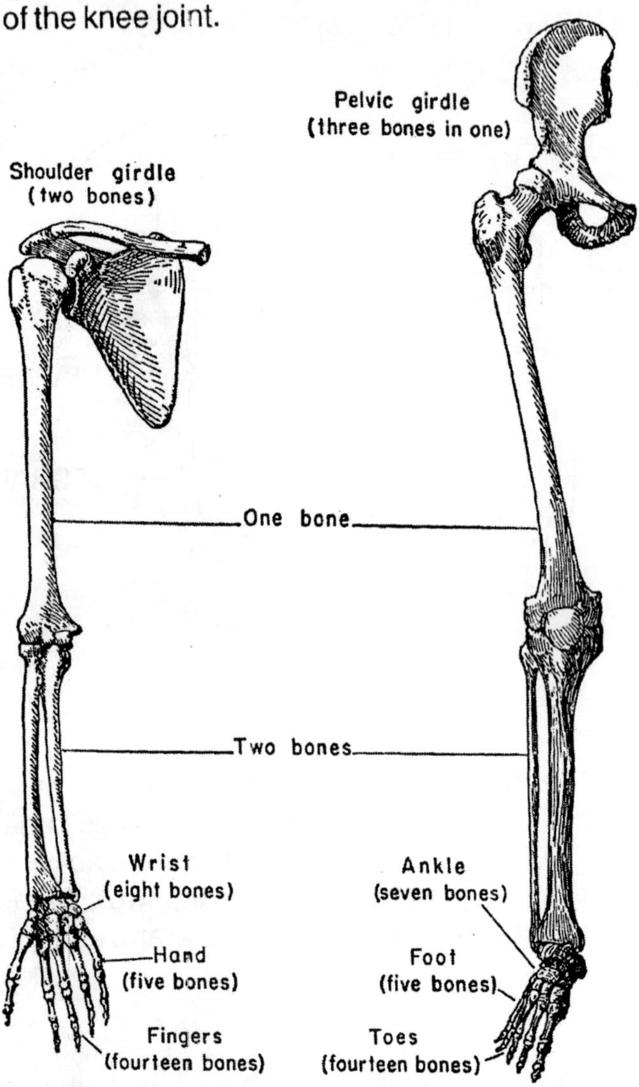

JOINTS AND LIGAMENTS

A joint formed where two bones come together. Some joint are immovable, like those in the skull. Bones are held together by ligaments, which are tough, white or yellow bands running between the bones and enclosing the joint. Ligaments are often partially torn in accidents. They heal slowly.

MUSCLES AND TENDONS

The red flesh covering the skeleton consists mostly of muscle. There are many muscle in the body. Each one has the ability to shorten itself when it gets a nerve impulse from the brain or spinal cord.

Most muscles are attached at each end to bones, either directly or by means of strong, white cords called tendons. When a muscle shortens, it produces movement by pulling upon the bone to which it is fastened.

SIMPLE AND COMPOUND FRACTURES

A break in a bone is called a fracture. Most fractures result from automobile accident and falls. Bullets often cause fracture when they strike bones.

Fractures are of two main kinds, compound and simple. In a compound fracture there is, in addition to the broken bone, a wound extending from the break through the skin. This wound may have been caused if a bullet or other object went through the skin and broke the bone; or the wound may have been caused if one of the bone ends protruded at least temporarily through the skin. In a simple fracture a wound extending thorough the skin is not present. Compound fractures are especially bad because germs are carried deep into the flesh around the broken ends, and an infection is likely to develop there. Simple fractures are bad enough, but with them an infection is much less likely.

If a person with simple fracture is handled or transported without proper care, a broken end may pierce the skin, making the simple fracture a compound fracture. This may also occur if a person with a broken leg tries to walk. Mishandling a simple fracture so that it becomes compound is a grave error in first aid.

ESTIMATING BLOOD LOSS BY SITE AND NUMBER OF FRACTURES

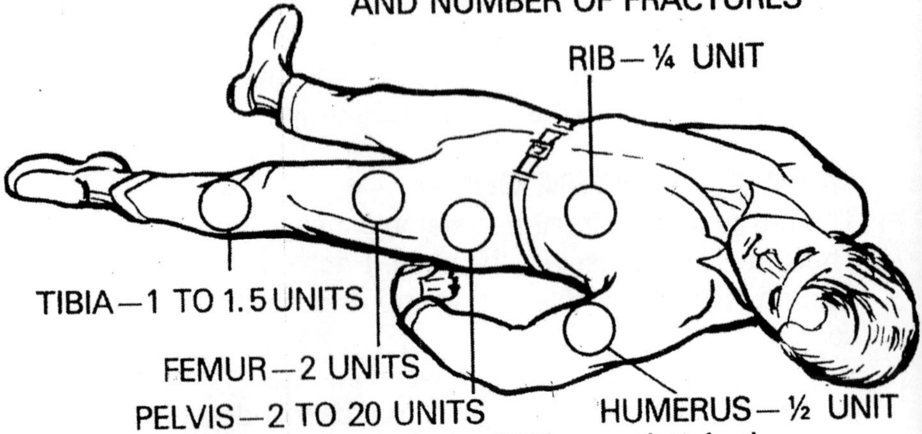

Fracture bleeding will usually be 50% complete in the first 4 to 6 hours.

THE MOST SEVERE BLOOD LOSS OCCURS IN FRACTURE OF THE PELVIS

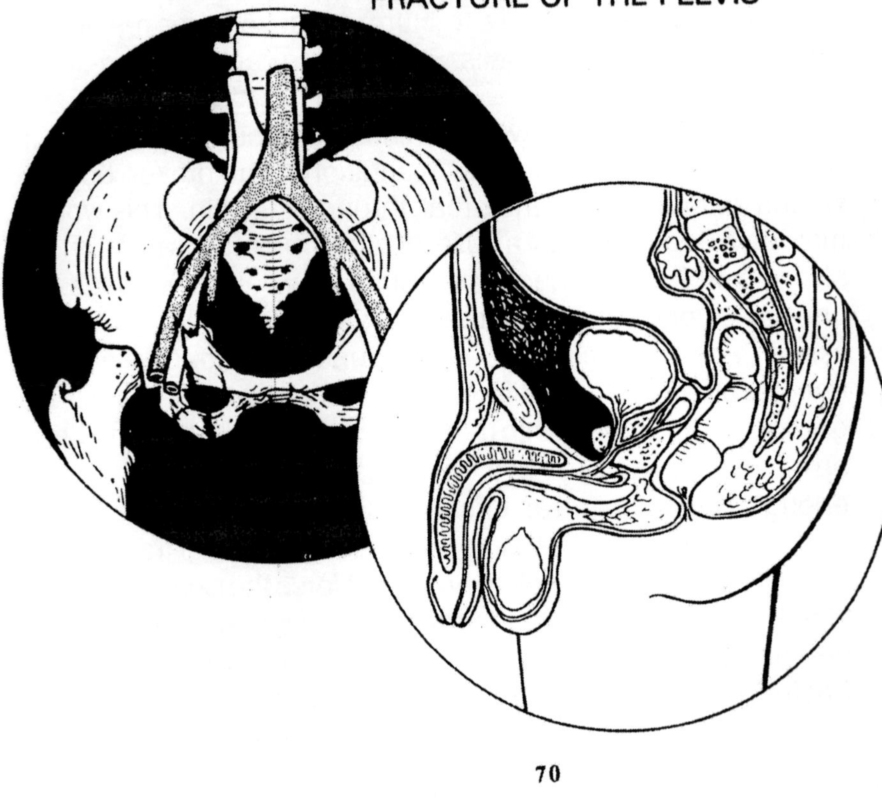

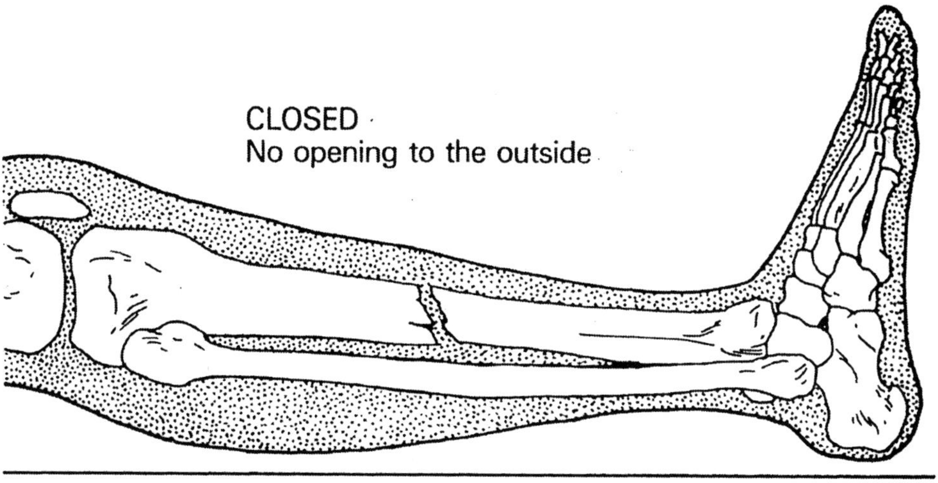

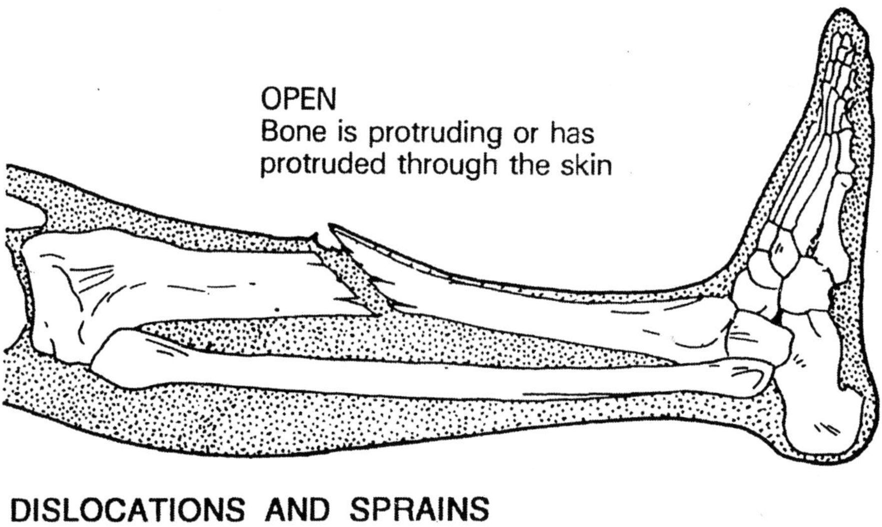

DISLOCATIONS AND SPRAINS

DISLOCATIONS

Because of a fall or blow, a bone may be dislocated, that is, sprung out of place at a joint. The signs are almost like those for a fracture. One usually cannot tell except by X-ray whether a bone is dislocated or broken. You should therefore give first aid in the same way as already described for a fracture.

SPRAINS

Sprains sometimes occur when there is great pressure on the bones and surrounding flesh at joint. For instance, when a person

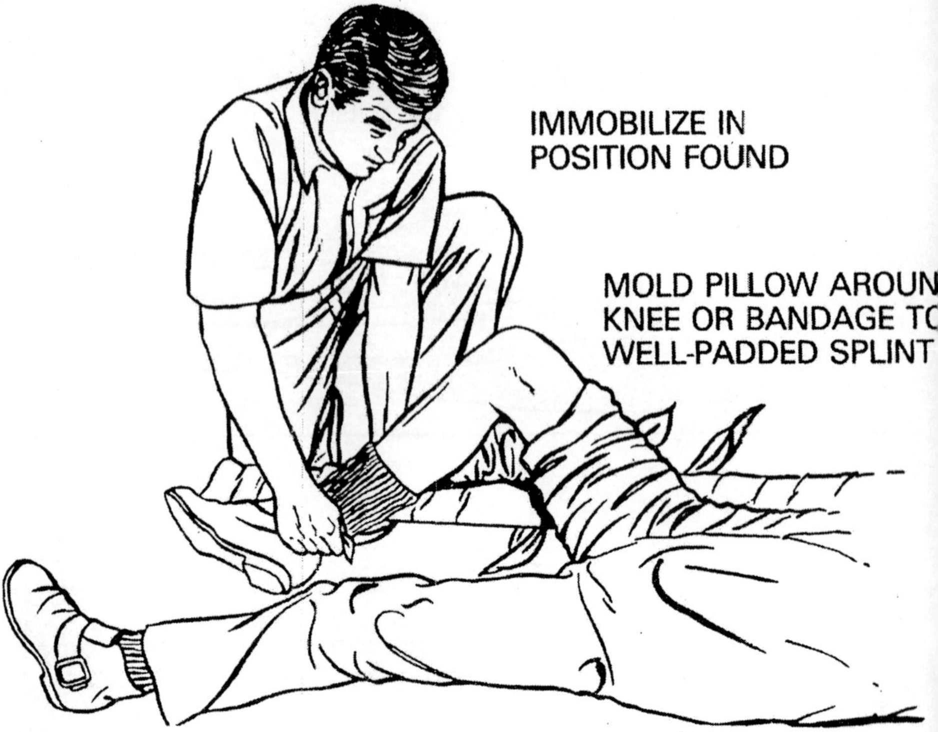
IMMOBILIZE IN
POSITION FOUND
MOLD PILLOW AROUN
KNEE OR BANDAGE T
WELL-PADDED SPLINT

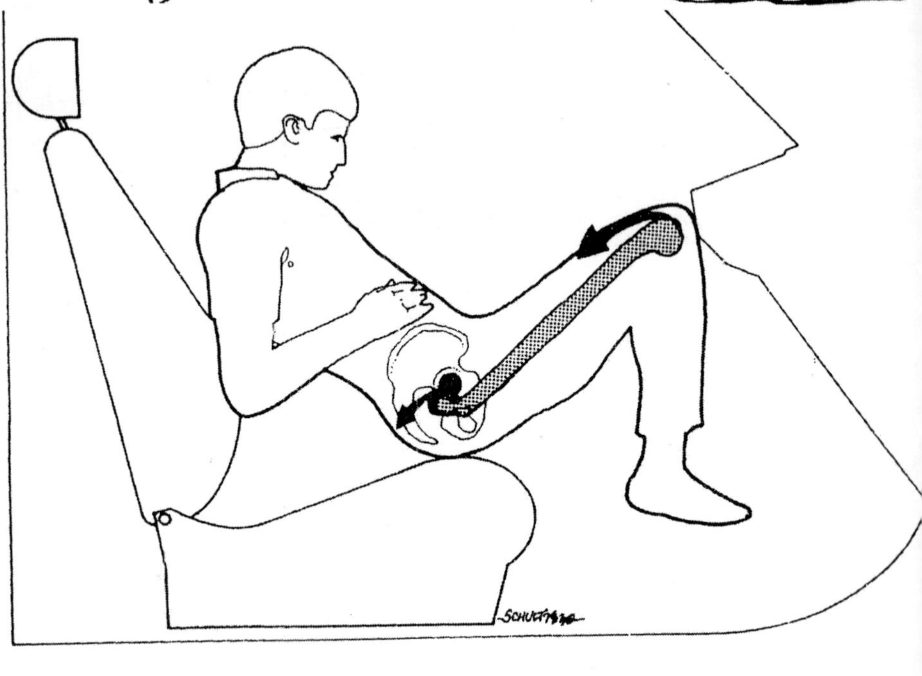

twist his foot, he put much strain on the ankle joint. In case of sprain the bone does not spring out of place or break, but the flesh around the joint (ligaments, muscle, and tendons) is stretched or even torn somewhat.

Pain is present at first, then swelling and perhaps discoloration. The commonest sprains occur at the ankle and the wrist.

Since one cannot be sure whether the injury is a sprain or a fracture, X-ray is always advisable. Sometimes people with ankle fractures are wrongly permitted to walk because the first aider thinks the injury is a sprain. Even in sprain cases it is best not to walk until the doctor advises it.

Clothes wet with cold water should be applied to a sprain, the sooner after injury the better. Cold cloths do not have nearly so much value if their application is delayed even 15 minutes. The cold applications may be continued a half hour or longer. The injured part should be kept quiet. It is best for the victim to lie down, with the injured part elevated somewhat on a pillow or other support. The doctor may advise that warm applications be applied later on, or he may tape the ankle.

CHEST INJURIES

Anatomy

The thorax is a bony sage that encloses the following:

1. Heart
2. Lungs
3. Aorta
4. Superior and inferior vena cava
5. Trachea and bronchi
6. Esophagus
7. Diaphragm
8. Spinal cord

Also lying within the bounds of the rib cage are the

1. Kidneys
2. Spleen
3. Liver
4. Pancreas
5. Stomach

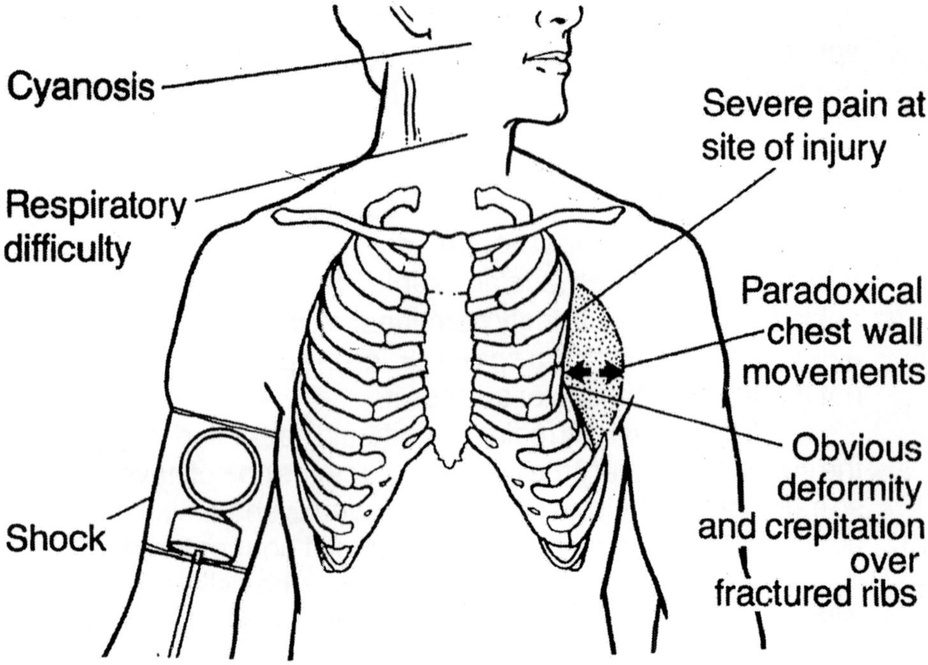

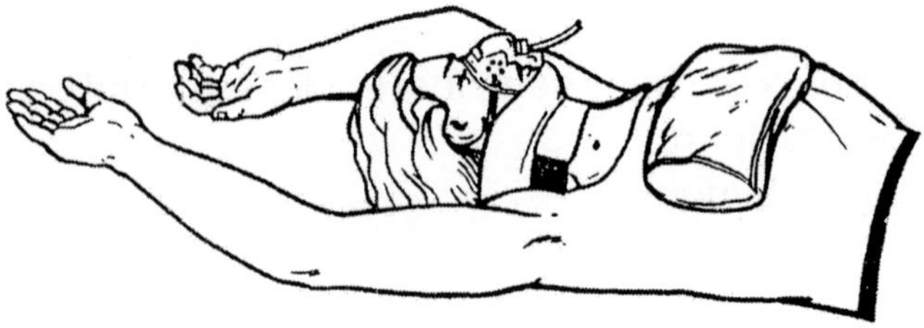

STABILIZE FLAIL SECTION BY APPLYING SANDBAG

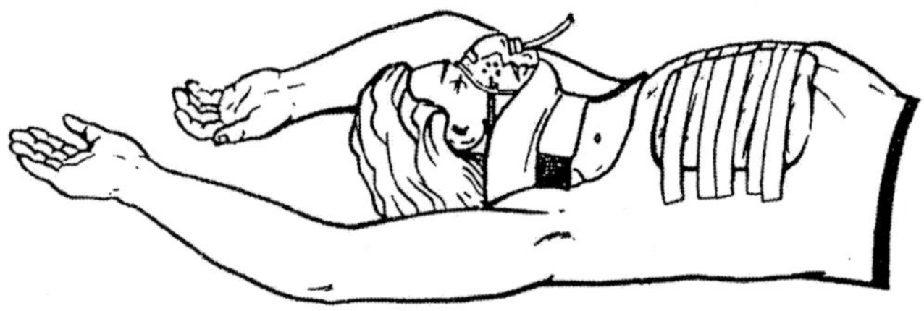

TAPE PAD IN PLACE, EXTENDING TAPE TO BOTH SIDES OF CHEST

Thus, trauma to the body in the area covered by the rib cage can injure any one or several of the structures listed. Here again, you must be alert to the history and the scene of the accident in order to think of mechanisms of injury. Then a careful, systematic evaluation, keeping in mind the possible injuries, must be made.

Pathophysiology

When you are evaluating a victim, always think of the most dangerous injuries first so as to give your patient the greatest chance for survival. If you do a great job splinting an ankle but your patient dies of an airway obstruction, you will never develop the reputation of a lifesaver.

Injuries Capable of Producing Death Within a Few Moments

A.Airway obstruction

1. Evaluation of the airway is always the first priority in evaluating any patient. You must look, listen, and feel for movement of air.
2. If the victim is making respiratory effort but no air is moving or if he is making no respiratory effort, the airway must be opened immediately. Do not forget to stabilize the cervical spine while gaining control of the airway.

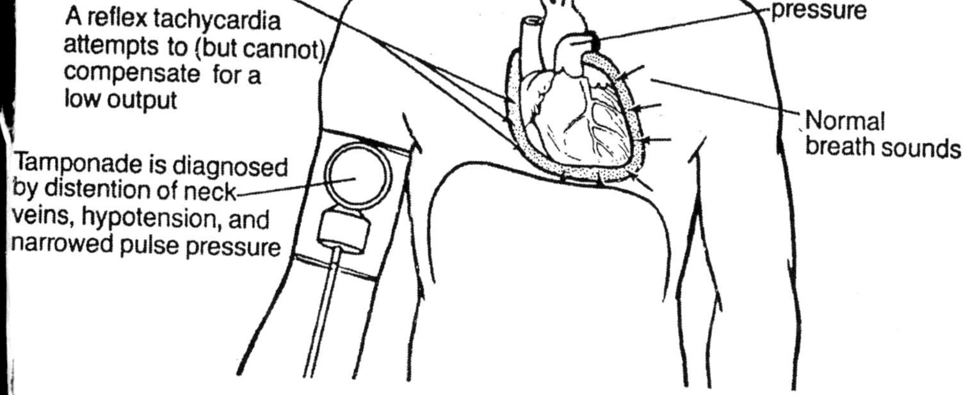

B. Open pneumothorax (sucking chest wound)

1. Pathophysiology: Normally, the chest expands and the diaphragm contacts causing a negative pressure inside the chest. Air rushes in through the upper airway and trachea and expands the lungs. When the diaphragm and chest relax, a positive pressure is formed that forces the air back out the same route. If the chest sustains a penetrating injury (e.g., knife or missile) large enough to remain open, air will enter and exit the chest with the change in intrathoracic pressure; however, this air will only enter the pleural space (causing the lung to collapse). It will not enter the lung and therefore will not contribute to oxygenation of the blood. Air will follow the path of least resistance, so if the opening is larger than the glottic opening, more air will enter the pleural pace than the lungs. In other words, the movement of the ribs and diaphragm will be unable to form enough negative pressure to ventilate the lungs, and the victim will smother as surely as if he had an airway obstruction.
2. Diagnosis of sucking chest wound: There is generally no difficulty with this diagnosis. The patient will have sustained some sort of penetrating trauma to the chest, he will have trouble moving air even though his airway is open, and, generally, he will have another opening in the chest that you can both see and hear.
3. Treatment of sucking chest wound:

A. Close the wound: This can be done with anything that will seal the wound. Have the patient exhale just before you seal the opening. A gel defibrillator pad (Littman, 3M) works best because it will stick to wet or dry skin. Petrolatum gauze or Saran TM wrap also works well. For larger wounds, a thin rubber glove with the tip of a finger cut off can be used in the same manner. However, time is so important in this situation that the simpler procedure (defibrillator pad or Saran wrap) is better.

B. Give oxygen.

C. If there is no danger of spinal injury (stab wound only), you may transport the victim on the affected side. This allows the uninjured lung to function best. If there is any danger of spinal injury, the victim must be transported supine on a spine board with neck stabilized.

References

Anderson, M.B.; and Williams, J.M. (1988) A model of stress and athletics injury: Prediction and prevention. Journal of sport and Exercise Psychology. 10,294-306.

Andrews, J.R.; and Gillogly, S. (1985) Physical examination of the shoulder in throwing athletes. In Zarins, B; Andrews, J.R.; and Carson, W.G. (Eds) Injuries to the Throwing Arm. Philadelphia: W.B. Saunders Co.

Arno, S.(1990) The A angle : A quantitative measurement of patella alignment and realignment. J. of Orthopaedic and Sports Physical Therapy. 12,6237-242.

Bandura, A.(1982) Self efficacy mechanism in human agency. American Psychologists, 37,122-14.

Balysis, W.J.; and Rzonca, E.C. (1988) Common sports injuries to the knee. Clinics in Podiatric Medicine and Surgery, 5,3.

Bearden, J.M.; Hughston, J.C.; and Whatley, G.S. (1973) Acromioclavicular dislocation : Method of treatment. J. of sports Med. 1,5.

Beecker, H.K. (1959) Measurement of Subjective Responses, Oxford University Press, Oxford.

Bodnar, L.M. (1977) Sports medicine with reference to back and neck injuries. Curr. Prect. Orthop. Surg., 7,116-153.

Booth, R.E. Jr.; and Marvel, J.P. Jr. (1975) Differential diagnosis of shoulder pain. Orthop. Clin North. Am., 6,353.

Bramwell, S.; Masuda, M.; Wagner, N.; and Holmes, T. (1975)

Psychological factors in athletic injuries. J. of Human Stress, 1, 6-20.

Cantu, R.C. (1987) Head and cervical spine injuries. In Cantu, R.C. (Ed.) The Exercising Adult. New York: Mac Millan Publishing Co.

Coddington, R.; and Troxell, T. (1980) The effects of emotional factors on football injury rates- a pilot study. J. of Human stress, 6, 3-5.

Cox, A.J. (1990) Biomechanics of the patello-femoral joint. Clinical Biomechanics, 5, 123-130.

Crossman, J.; Jamieson, j.; and Henderson, L. (1987) Responses of competitive athletes to lay-offs in training : Exercise addiction or psychological relief ? Jounal of Sport Behaviour, 10, (1), 28-38.

Exler, Y. (1991) Patella facture : Review of the litrature and five case presentations. J. of Orthopaedic and Sports Physical Therapy, 13,4,177-183.

Eysenck, H.J. (1957) The Dynamics Anxiety and Hysteria. London: Routledge and Kogan Paul.

Eysenck, H.J. (1967) The Biological Basis of Personality.Illinois: C.C. Thomas, Springfield.

Garrick, J.G.; and Webb, D.R. (1990) Sports Injuries : Diagnosis and Management. London : W.B. Saunders.

Gordon, S.; Milios, D.; and Grove, J.R. (1991) Psychological aspects of the recovery process from sport injury : The perspective of sport physiotherapists. Australian Journal of Science and Medicine in Sport, 23, (2), 53-60.

Griffiths, D. (1980) Psychology and Medicine. London: Mac Millan.

Harari, H. (1969) Levels of aspirations and athletic performance. Perceptual and Motor Skills, 28, 519-524.

Henning, C.E. (1988) Semilunar cartilage of the knee : Function and pathology. Exercise and Sports Science Review, 16, 205-213.

Heppenstall, R.B. (1975) Fractures and dislocations of the distal clavicle. Orthop. Clin. North. Am., 6,477.

Hutson, M.A. (1996) Prevention of injury. In Hutson, M.A. (Ed) Sports Injuries : Recognision and Management. Oxford : Oxford University Press.

Jackson, D. W.; Jarrett, H.; Bailey, D.; Kausek, J.; Swanson, J.; and Powell, J.W. (1978) Injury prediction in the young athlete : A preliminary report. American, J. of Sports Medicine, 6,6-14.

Jerosch, J.G.; Castro, W.H.M.; and Jantea, C. (1989) Stress fracture of the patella. American J. of sports Medicine, 17,4.

Kelley, M.J. (1990) Meniscal trauna (of the knee) and surgical intervention. J. of Sports Medicine and Physical Fitness, 30, 3, 297-306.

Kerr, G.; and Minden, H. (1988) Psychological factors related to the occurrence of athletic injuries. J. of sports Psycholog.

Lewthwaite, R. (1990) Motivational considerations in physical activity involvement. Physical Therapy, 70 (12), 808-819.

Locke, E.A.; and Bryan, J.F. (1966) Cognitive aspects of psychomotor performance: The effects of performance goals on levels of performance. Journal of Applied Psychology, 50, 286-291.

Mcleod, W.D. (1985) The pitching mechanism. In zarins, B.;

Andrews, J.R.; and Carson, W.G. (Eds). Injuries to the Throwing Arm. Philadelphia : W.B. Sauders Co.

Mehlhoff, T.L.; Noble, P.C.; Bennett, J.B.; and Tullos, H.S. (1988) Simple dislocation of the elbow in the adult : Results after closed treatment. J. of Bone and Joint Surgery, 70A, 244-249.

Nigg, B.M. (1988) The assessment of loads acting on the locomotor system in running and other sport activities. Seminars in Orthopaedics, 4(3), 197-206.

Norris, C.M. (1993) Sports Injuries : Diagnosis and Management for Physiotherapists. Oxford: Butterworth-Heinemann.

Noyes, F.R.; Bassett, R.W.; Grood, E.S.; and Butler, D.L. (1980) Arthroscopy in acute traumatic haemarthrosis of the knee. J. of Bone Joint Surgery, 62A, 687-95.

Palastange, N.; Field, D.; and Soames, R. (1989) Anatomy and Human Movement, Oxford : Heinemann Medical.

Reilly, T. (1975) An Ergonomic Evaluation of Occupational Stress in Professional Football. Doctoral Thesis, Liverpool Polytechnic.

Rowe, C.R.; and Zarins, B. (1981) Recurrent transient subluxation of the shoulder. J. of Bone Joint Surg. 63A, 863.

Rowe, C.R.; and Zarins, B.(1982) Chronic unreduced dislocations of the shoulder. J. of Bone Joint Surg., 64A, 494.

Sanderson, F.H. (1977) The psychology of the injury-prone athlete. British Journal of Sports Medicine, 11, 56-57.

Sanderson, F.H. (1981) The psychology of injur-prone athlete. In Reilly, T. (Ed,) Sports Fitness and sports Injuries. London: Faber and Faber.

Scott, D.; Bird, H.A.; and Wright, V. (1979) Joint laxity leading to osteoarthrosis. Rheum. Rehabil. 18, 167-169.

Shields, C.L., Jr.; Fox, J.M.; and Stauffer, E.S. (1978) Cervical cord injuries in sports. Phys. Sports Med., 6, 71-76.

Simonet, W.T.; and Cofield, R.H. (1984) Prognosis in anterior shoulder dislocation. Am. J. of Sports Med., 12,19.

Speakman, H.G.B.; and Weisberg, J. (1977) The vastus medialis controversy. Physiotherapy, 63, 8, 249-254.

Taimela, S.; Kujala, UM.; and Osterman, K. (1990) Intrinsic risk factors and athletic injuries. Sports Medicine, 9(4), 205-215.

Torg, J.S. (1989) In year Book of sports Medicine (ed. R.J. Shephard, J.L. Anderson, E.R. Eichner et al.) Chicago : Yearbook Medical Publishers, p.186.

Watkins, J.(1983) An Introduction to Mechanics of Human Movement, Lancaster: MTP Press.

Weiss, C.B.; Lundberg, M.; Hamberg, P.: Dettaven, K.E.; and Gillquist, J. (1989) Non-operative treatment of meniscal tears. J. of Bone and Joint Surgery, 71A, 811-822.

Williams, J.G.P. and Sperryn, P.N. (1976) Sports Medicine, London : Edward Arnold.

Williams, J.I. (1989) Illness behaviour to wellness behaviour. Physiotherapy, 75, (1), 2-7.